The ADHD Women's Wellbeing *Toolkit*

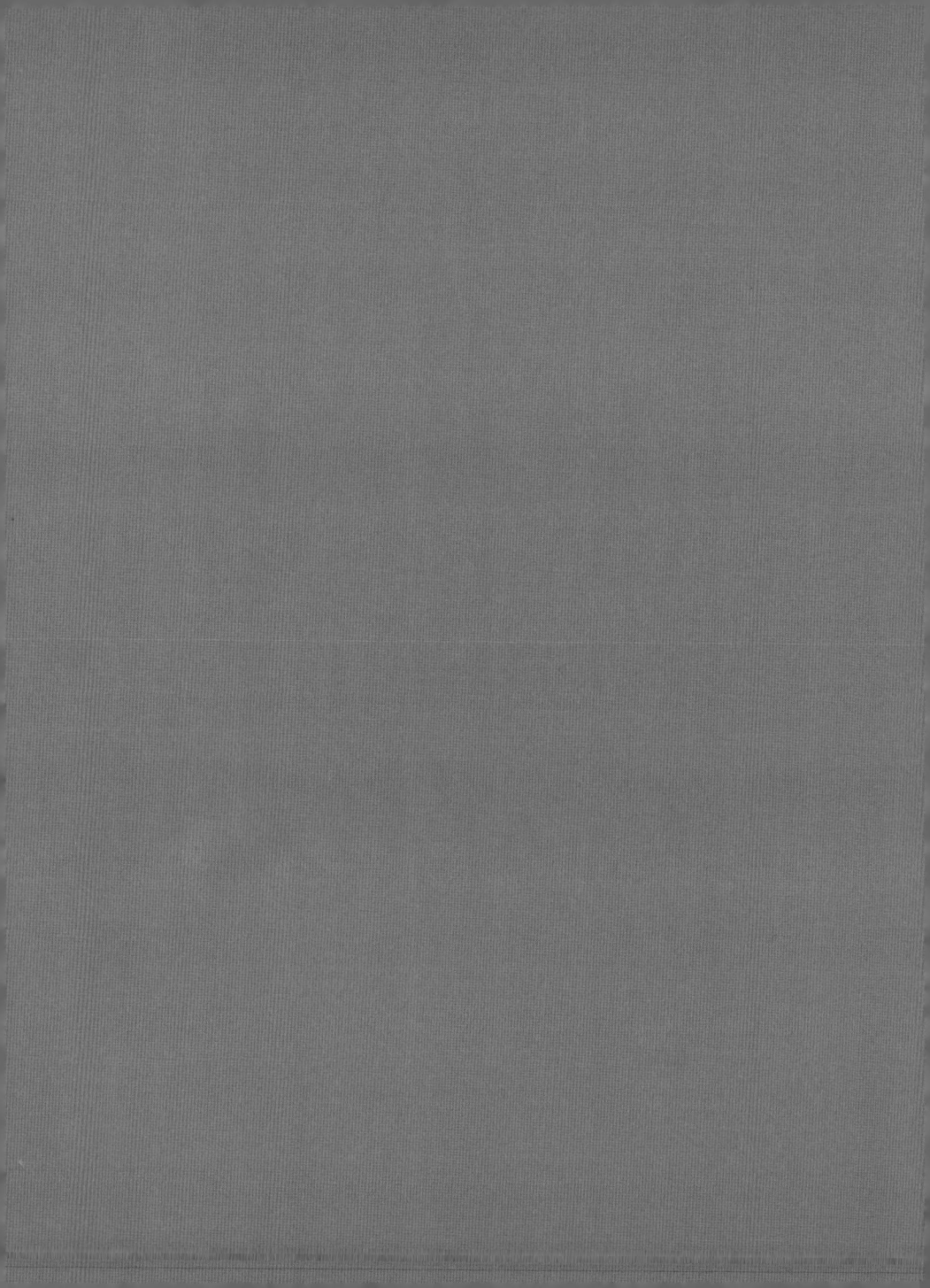

KATE MORYOUSSEF

The ADHD Women's Wellbeing Toolkit

Embrace your authentic self
and harness your true potential

DK [RED]

Advance praise for

The ADHD Women's Wellbeing Toolkit

'Relevant and practical. This book is going to be so helpful and empowering to so many women!'
Dr Lotta Borg Skogland, M.D., Ph.D., author and psychiatrist

'Seamlessly integrates the latest scientific understanding of the brain and the practical approaches that can lead to a fulfilling life for a woman with ADHD.'
Sari Solden, MS, ADHD expert, psychotherapist, and author

'A compassionate companion for every woman seeking to transform overwhelm into empowerment.'
Dr Miguel Toribio-Mateas, clinical neuroscientist

'A treasure trove of resources to cultivate understanding, acceptance, and practical ways of navigating life with ADHD.'

Suzy Reading, author and chartered psychologist

'Finally, a brilliant toolkit for women living with ADHD to help them thrive rather than just survive.'

Lucinda Miller, author and clinical lead of NatureDoc

'I will be telling many of my patients about this book.'

Dr Ruth Verrier Jones, GP

Contents

Introduction

How are you feeling? *Really* feeling? Living most of your adult life with undiagnosed Attention Deficit Hyperactivity Disorder (ADHD) can feel like walking around in the wrong shoes while carrying a backpack full of rocks, wondering why you're finding things tough. It can be soul-destroying, and it can burn you out. I believe there is a better way, a more hopeful way. In fact, that's exactly what this book is about. But first, we need to look at how we got here.

ADHD in women

Until quite recently, ADHD was mostly overlooked in girls and women. Only a handful of women were diagnosed in childhood; most were diagnosed, like me, later on in life. From the late 1980s, ADHD (or ADD, Attention Deficit Disorder, as it was then known) was seen as something that only affected young boys, with the leading trait being that they couldn't, or wouldn't, sit still at school. They were dismissed as disruptive, disinterested, and naughty. Many of their stories are heartbreaking.

What we have come to understand in recent years is that ADHD in females can look very different from ADHD in males. For girls and women, hyperactive traits are often internalised (and frequently diagnosed as anxiety and/ or depression) because of traditional gender conditioning. Hormones also have a role to play in how and when ADHD expresses itself. While some females do display some of the rambunctious traits we often see in males, we now understand that ADHD can show up for them in a variety of other ways. This might include perfectionism, insomnia, forgetfulness, disorganisation, daydreaming, overthinking, restlessness, overwhelm, emotional dysregulation, mood swings, and a quiet lack of concentration.

The stereotype of what ADHD is 'meant to' look like means that ADHD traits in women and girls have been misunderstood and under-researched for far too long. It's vital that the many nuanced symptoms and traits of ADHD expression in girls and women are recognised as such, so that health and education professionals can look out for these, ask more questions, and start to connect the dots in order to provide more support.

Beginning a journey of understanding

As things stand, the study of ADHD in females still lacks significant scientific and medical evidence in comparison to its study in males,[1] while medical professionals focus their research on how ADHD coexists with autism, dyslexia, dysgraphia, dyscalculia, and dyspraxia. A lot of what I know and share in this book comes from playing detective through my various roles as host of *The ADHD Women's Wellbeing Podcast*, an accredited Emotional Freedom Technique (EFT) practitioner, and health and wellbeing coach. Through the podcast, I am able to speak to hundreds of leading experts and thought leaders in the field of ADHD who share their knowledge with our listeners – a strong community of women who are self-diagnosed or formally diagnosed with ADHD.

This knowledge helps us begin to draw our own conclusions about ADHD and its impact. We are only at the beginning of this journey, but I hope that this book will allow you to gain new insights, better understanding, more practical tools, and lots of self-compassion, so that you can begin thriving and enjoying a better quality of life. Importantly, I hope that you can feel a part of this growing community of brilliant women with ADHD.

You deserve to experience kindness from others and, most importantly, from yourself.

The importance of self-acceptance

When I work with clients who are living with ADHD, I can see their desperation to be 'fixed'. But I want to tell you right here and now, as I was myself told, that you do not need 'fixing'. The challenges we face are not our fault; they are rooted in our genes, in our biology, and are – importantly – neurological. You're not lazy, stupid, rude, strange, scatty, or selfish: you have ADHD with neurodivergent brain wiring, which can have a daily impact on your mental and physical health.

Even if you don't feel it yet, you are completely brilliant. And this book is here to show you how to lean into your cognitive capabilities, finally let go of all the conditioning – the shoulds, needs, and ought tos – and give yourself permission to thrive on your own terms.

We've been told all our lives that there's one linear (outdated!) way to get from A to B, but this simply isn't true. To put it plainly: you are allowed to be authentically you. You are allowed to live life more effortlessly and easily, and yes, this may look different to the path others are on, but different isn't wrong. It is time to set out on your own journey. Who knows where it will lead?

ADHD and me

Though we will be looking at many of the commonly held traits of women with ADHD, we all have unique journeys. For me personally, I never understood why I was so sensitive to stress, why my anxiety would show up at the smallest provocation, and why I would lose my rag like a four-year-old having a temper tantrum while others around me could remain so calm. I sensed a build-up of physical energy that I couldn't explain. I often had to get myself moving first thing in the morning and ideally again in the afternoon to successfully expel the building restlessness that other girls I knew just didn't have. My hyperactivity wasn't very easy to detect on the outside, but inwardly it felt like rising lava, ready to blow and destroy anyone in its wake.

My ADHD presented subtly, yet it still managed to impact my education and career. I could feel my brain ticking away, when all I wanted it to do was shut down and be quiet. It constantly created catastrophised 'what if' scenarios and played out the worst situations (especially at night) until my heart would pound and my tummy would hurt. I was still undiagnosed when my internalised anxiety, something that I only discovered in my 30s, caused me to develop Inflammatory Bowel Syndrome (IBS). I was given anti-nausea medication and told to avoid dairy. That was it. There was no discussion about the gut–brain connection and how stress and worry can impact our gut health and vice versa.

Awareness and diagnosis

My ADHD diagnosis itself came late, at the age of 40, alongside that of my then nine-year-old daughter. As I was helping her with homeschooling during the Covid pandemic, I noticed traits that I understood so well in myself were also showing up in her. Yet it was only when I read a short article on ADHD in girls that I knew it was what we were both dealing with.

Though our ADHD manifested differently – as is often the case – I knew I had to advocate strongly to get us both diagnoses. And it was from this moment of self-diagnosis that our lives really began to change. Initially there was grief, but soon after there was relief. I began to understand my own life better, and I also realised there would be millions of others just like me.

I'm now nearly five years post-diagnosis and I deeply understand how undiagnosed ADHD impacts women's lives, with symptoms ranging from an appalling lack of self-belief to feeling that we have underachieved throughout life. The continuous masking, overcompensating, doubting our abilities, and questioning of ourselves can lead to chronic exhaustion and ongoing burnout cycles. Studies have demonstrated that neurodivergent women are about 30% more likely to suffer from the emotional and physical exhaustion of burnout than neurotypical women.[2]

Recognising the symptoms

ADHD can affect our mental health too, contributing to crippling anxiety, low moods, depression, Obsessive Compulsive Disorder (OCD), insomnia, emotional dysregulation, irritability, and anger. Early research studies show that ADHD can be affected by female hormones, exacerbating symptoms of Premenstrual Dysphoric Disorder (PMDD), endometriosis, postnatal depression, and early perimenopause. It can also manifest in our bodies as stress-related conditions such as IBS, fibromyalgia, Chronic Fatigue Syndrome (CFS), thyroid issues, eczema, adrenal fatigue, chronic pain, migraines, and autoimmune conditions – although more research is needed to establish and prove the scientific links in all of these areas.[3]

I'd like to be able to tell you that once you have awareness of your ADHD it's all plain sailing; and yes, it can set you on the path to accessing better support (including medication, for those who want to go down this route), and the understanding it brings is hugely validating. However, we still have to learn how to manage every day, to process and eventually release the past, destress, regulate, and offer ourselves and those around us more compassion and forgiveness. We can then lean in and allow our ever-resourceful brains to help us move forward and thrive. It is this process that I hope to help you with in the coming pages.

Whether you have a diagnosis or are just exploring the possibility of one, remember that you are enough.

How to use this book

This is a pick-and-mix toolkit curated to help you with the often daily challenges you may face. It offers advice for different days and recognises that at varying stages in your life you will need different things: sometimes you will be thriving, sometimes struggling. It will show you the power you possess to make choices and lifestyle changes that will help you, and that you can live in the present without anxiety and fear. Whether you are reading this book for yourself or a loved one, you are sure to find lots of actionable ideas for how to better support yourself or someone else with ADHD. Although this book focuses on ADHD in those assigned female at birth, it is designed to benefit anyone who is living with ADHD or suspects that they might have it, regardless of their gender.

You can open the book at any page and dive in, but I have also written it as a roadmap to uncovering your authentic self, whether that's before or after diagnosis. It explores why we behave and think as we do with our ADHD brains, delving into the issues we face and offering solutions and tools to help.

Each chapter outlines a problem that we face or a goal to achieve, before breaking things down in more detail. We then identify the scaffolding to build you up and what we can do to make it better, introducing specific tools to help us get there. Not every tool will be right for everyone at every time, but by providing a range of ADHD-tailored advice, you can find what works for you. You'll also be able to read expert opinions from leading thinkers and researchers in the field and insights from real women with ADHD. I've added reflective moments and prompts too, to help you make the most of your unique journey.

More than anything, I hope the following guidance will help you to convince your brain that it is okay and safe to be present. The day-by-day tweaking and updating of thoughts, behaviours, and habits alongside a true understanding of ADHD will set you on the right path and help you to feel happier overall. It is time to understand your past, accept your present, and learn how to light up your future.

CHAPTER 1

Awaken Who You Uniquely Are

Before we dive into specific symptoms of living with ADHD, let's take time to build a strong foundation for our learning. In this chapter, we'll examine what ADHD is and how it affects us as individuals, the highs and the lows, and explore how we can start to move towards self-acceptance.

What does it mean to have ADHD?

There is no one-size-fits-all interpretation when it comes to ADHD. While it may be easy to define on paper, the lived experience will feel very different for everyone.

ADHD is neurodevelopmental, which means it is related to the development of our brain and nervous system. It is understood to have a genetic component[4] and to be influenced by external stressors. Historic testing for ADHD states that the condition can present in different ways: usually hyperactivity, impulsivity, and inattention, or a combination of all three (but this is a very binary way of looking at a complex issue). Each of these impacts on our ability to live calm, happy lives.

Though scientific explanations are helpful, they are only half of the story. So what does the lived experience of ADHD actually *feel* like? ADHD will feel different for everyone, but struggles include feeling overwhelmed and anxious. Sadly, signs often go unnoticed in women because we have been conditioned to mask them. It is common for ADHD women to be told, 'you always look so put-together', when all we want to do is scream, 'I have created manic coping mechanisms, just to ensure that I don't drop a ball, lose a child, or end up fired from my job!'

It can be exhausting, draining, and depleting, causing many burnout cycles and health crises. We may have been dismissed by our doctors and prescribed medication that only scratches the surface, all while innately knowing that something else, quite devastating, is going on within our brains and bodies.

CO-EXISTING CONDITIONS

ADHD can often co-occur with other conditions, such as autism (many identify as AuDHD), OCD, depression, anxiety, bi-polar disorder, dyslexia, dyscalculia, disordered eating, and addiction.

Getting diagnosed

Having an ADHD diagnosis can be life-changing for many women, and it was for me. When I was diagnosed, I felt such a polarity of emotions. However, despite all this, I was no longer questioning why I behaved, worked, felt, and acted the way I did.

If you don't have a formal diagnosis and would like to seek one, make an appointment with your doctor to talk through the process. Go to that meeting ready to advocate for yourself and explain why you feel you have ADHD. Hopefully you'll speak to someone well-informed and empathetic, who gives support and advice; remember that you can always ask for a second opinion. And don't forget that the ADHD community will always listen and help. Here in the UK, the NHS waiting lists are so long that many of us are seeking private diagnoses, which are just as valid.

Post-diagnosis, any given day could bring a whirlwind of emotions: elated, overwhelmed, exhausted, grateful, angry, accepting, ashamed, and excited. As I was navigating my own story, it transpired that so many other women across the world were living similar lives.

I decided to find out everything I could about ADHD to help myself, my children, and the numerous women I now support daily. It's only with increased awareness that we're finally given the tools to build a life with structures that work *for* us, and not against us. This includes setting new boundaries and rediscovering the world according to our needs. And wow, there is a whole new territory to explore.

IN HER SHOES

An ADHD diagnosis has been life-changing... I am much kinder to myself, more accepting of my challenges, and am leaning into my strengths.

Ornitha, 49

The importance of a diagnosis

DR HANNAH CULLEN, counselling psychologist specialising in assessment and treatment for adult ADHD

> *To witness the shift in a client who has just been diagnosed with ADHD will always be a remarkable moment in my work. One of my favourite responses was from a client in her mid-30s who upon receiving her diagnosis of ADHD declared 'It's like a light has finally been switched on in a dark room.'*
>
> *While this moment of clarity and relief is often profound, it is soon met with a multitude of emotions at once, and so, we then dance with grief. There is a pain that runs deeply in clients who have been diagnosed late in life. There can be a tremendous sense of loss in that perhaps life somehow would have been so different; easier.*
>
> *Many of my clients have experienced significant rejection for most of their lives, and report 'feeling different to others'. When growing up, most were shamed, often told they were 'too sensitive', 'too loud', 'too angry', 'too messy', or even 'stupid'. This shapes the internal voice of that child and how they then navigate the world as an adult. The harsh and critical inner dialogue of a client living undiagnosed with ADHD adds to their experience of self-blame, self-criticism, and excessive worry.*
>
> *Carving out a safe and gentle space for a client to feel these difficult emotions is one of the most important aspects of healing for an adult who receives an ADHD diagnosis. Often, a lifetime has been spent actively avoiding processing the pain of shame, loneliness, disconnect, and trauma. Addiction, humour, or self-harm often swoop in to temporarily help us cope, so we don't have to feel a deeper pain. But it is just that, temporary; we must go there in order to leave there.*
>
> *With the right therapeutic support, a client can learn to change their inner dialogue and finally meet so many of their unmet needs. This monumental shift in self-love, self-acceptance, and validation is when a client begins to flourish and thrive.*

The challenges of ADHD

There can be many advantages to living with ADHD, but we will start by looking at some of the common challenges. Of course, ADHD isn't a box-ticking exercise, and not everything in the next sections will be relevant to you.

Forgive me for using headings that all begin with 'p' for this part – a quirk of my own ADHD hyperfocus in action! I thought that, if I'm going to encourage you to lean into all your idiosyncrasies and embrace them, then I should really follow the same advice and put my own ADHD personality and logic on display.

Perfectionism

This is often compounded by a lack of self-trust, fear of missing something, inattention, and imposter syndrome – all of which shout at you most days. You spend hours longer than needed on projects 'just in case'. Perfectionism leads to burnout, anxiety, and magnifies some OCD traits. Perfectionism stops us from being courageous when we want to change course or speak our truth.

Policing our thoughts

Oversharing and impulsivity are traits we often see in people with ADHD. They can be beneficial in many areas of our life – like helping us to connect to like-minded people. However, when we're not safe in our tribe, we can worry that we're going to say something we shouldn't. We end up overcompensating emotionally, masking, and not showing up as our authentic selves. We can't connect, and it feels awful and exhausting. Understanding this helps us to choose our friends discerningly and no longer try to be someone we aren't, freeing up our energy and time to live life more on our own terms.

People-pleasing

This stems from feeling like we're never quite fitting in, knowing that our brains work in their own way, or realising that we often think and behave differently from society's expectations. Yet we just keep on trying harder; we relinquish our own needs and put ourselves and our boundaries at the bottom of the pile.

Procrastination

Often, the only way many of us can begin a project is through last-minute adrenaline and fear, which over time takes its toll on us both mentally and physically while creating cycles of shame. When we begin to understand our working memory, executive functioning skills, dopamine response, and how we respond to pressure, we can find structures and strategies to cope better.

Pressure

The pressure we put on ourselves! Just because we have 96 ideas a day, it doesn't mean we need to implement them all at the same time. ADHD women can have a lot of drive, and this is a good thing! Perfectionism can also drive the internal pressure we put on ourselves. But our energy levels simply cannot match what goes on in our brains. We need more downtime to help offset our endless and exhausting internal motor.

Panic

Panic (and palpitations) can come from procrastination and pressure, combined with our mental processing and working memory differences. Panic impacts our stress response, sending us into a state of adrenaline-fuelled hypervigilance (often trauma-related), and putting our nervous system into fight-or-flight (known as 'sympathetic') mode.

IN HER SHOES

A lot of the challenge is in trying to explain to others how serious ADHD can be and how it affects nearly every area of your life. I struggle with how exhausted I get when I do anything remotely social, and with how much time I need to recharge.

Allie, 41

The joys of ADHD

While the challenges of ADHD can feel most prevalent, it's important to recognise some of the many ways in which an ADHD brain can bring joy and wonder to your life.

Powerful

I've reached the point where I know I'm working against the odds. Our successes are harder to achieve because of our neurodivergence. If that doesn't demonstrate that we're powerful and capable of many things, I don't know what does.

Persistent

For many of us, when we get ideas in our heads, there's no stopping us. We are tenacious and will seek answers, no matter how long it takes (even if our battery signs are flashing empty). Combine this with our deep desire for justice, especially advocating for what we're passionate about, and we are often the movers and shakers instilling big change in our communities.

Persuasive

If we decide we want to convince you of our plans, you're not going to escape! All of that hyperfocus and research can be channelled towards making our point and convincing others to come along for the ride.

Pure

There's an honesty and straightforwardness to our traits, which makes us authentic in a way that isn't often found elsewhere. We can be too trusting and be taken advantage of, and our strong moral compass may cause disappointment when others don't play by a similar rule book. We tend to accept people at face value (reserving all doubt and analysis for ourselves) and assume that *we're* the problem, not the world around us.

Passionate

Sometimes our single-mindedness can be a fantastic tool to effect change. When we really care about something, we're going to get stuck in and do our absolute best. We also love and care powerfully, and feel pain and rejection just as deeply.

Perceptive

We can be highly sensitive empaths, great at spotting problems that others don't see. The hypervigilance that can overwhelm our systems can also make us acutely aware of what's going on around us. We're trend-spotters, innovators, and entrepreneurs, creating new markets and niches and leading with an intuitive know-how that others can't explain.

Playful

Of course we are! We're fun, creative, and full of life. We have a wonderful, unique perspective on the world, and nothing thrills us more than channelling all of our energy into something we truly believe in. It may be fleeting, or it may last a decade, but when we're committed, we're all in; we find opportunities to be playful, inventive, and in flow with what we love to do.

Peculiar!

Finally, and I'll be the first to admit to this one, our ADHD idiosyncrasies are different for us all, but they make us the unique people we should also be proud of.

REFLECTIVE MOMENT

What are the positive parts of your ADHD experience? You might like to make some notes and keep them to hand, especially for when you're having a challenging day and may need some positive reminders of what you can achieve and how brilliant your brain often is.

Moving towards self-acceptance

Throughout this book we'll explore various aspects of the ADHD experience and you'll see how you can apply different tools to specific issues. Here is a short overview of the work we'll be doing, introducing some of the key tools we'll be applying.

Making peace with the present

Finding peace, forgiveness, and acceptance will set you on a path towards a more authentic and compassionate life. Some of this peace will come through practical exercises, such as prayers or mantras: these don't have to be religious; it's about taking the time to connect within, think about our needs, and what we are grateful for. Formulating these feelings into words and surrendering to a greater force, helps us recognise that we can't control it all and life suddenly feels lighter. Focused exercises will also allow you to practise being present, which is often not the default state for many of us. We'll look at how we can welcome small moments of mindfulness to feel more grounded.

Embracing who we are

We will also explore our curiosity to figure out what lights us up and how we can weave more agency into our lives. This may evolve as we get older, but having passion and being unapologetic about who we are will help us break free from shame. We need to find ways of believing in our potential, even when others don't. That means following our passions, even if they don't fall within the parameters of what others deem 'normal', and recognising what we're good at. We need to stop thinking, 'What if I cause a scene, make a stir, or rock the boat?' This is precisely what we're meant to do to create change.

Understanding the past

The relationship between trauma and ADHD is both complex and significant. While this book doesn't delve deeply into this topic, it's important to note that the connection is profound; I've yet to meet anyone in the ADHD space who hasn't been affected by trauma. ADHD is understood to have a genetic component and often runs in families, many of whom have been un/misdiagnosed, leaving generations without the tools and knowledge to navigate life effectively. Living in an undiagnosed neurodiverse family can lead to 'big T' traumas such as serious mental health conditions, parental dysfunction and chaos, addiction, divorce, suicide, and financial challenges. But we also often experience ongoing 'small T' traumas such as social rejection, financial struggle, imposter syndrome, masking, job insecurity, academic difficulties, or medical gaslighting. By recognising these painful traumatic moments and allowing ourselves time to heal, we're able to practise self-compassion, forgiveness, and empower ourselves for the future.

Creating conditions to flourish

We'll look at how to recognise and use tools that will help make life more managable, including asking for help, delegation, simplification, support, reflection, and organisation. We'll also examine how important it is to place ourselves in environments that help us lean into our strengths and flourish. We will assess our work situation, where we live, who we hang out with, what we eat, and how we move our bodies, with the aim of creating conditions that suit our skills, energy, and brains. What about when there's something we can't immediately fix? Well, sometimes we're just in a crappy situation, and we must recognise that and send ourselves compassion. We can use positive thinking, mantras, and affirmations to reframe our thoughts, rewire our brains, and lean into self-belief, resilience, and gratitude. We will discover how to harness new thoughts to get ourselves through difficult times and out the other side.

Next steps

We've clearly identified that, yes, ADHD can cause us difficulties day-to-day, but it also gifts us many wonderful skills and ways of looking at the world. The trick is to uncover an authentic lifestyle by employing strategies that allow us to manage the challenges we face while nurturing our talents, energy, and nervous system.

For me, gaining awareness of my ADHD has been one of the greatest gifts I've received. It has helped me find self-acceptance and discover tools and strategies to improve my life. I'm no longer afraid of my brain and I can see it for what it is. I am learning to be proud and compassionate towards my busy, innovative, curious, and empathic brain… most of the time.

I'm very much a work in progress, and suspect I will be for the rest of my days, learning, growing, evolving, failing, getting up, brushing myself off and, hopefully, inspiring others to do the same.

Acknowledge where you are

I can imagine that you also have mixed feelings about your own journey with ADHD, and I truly believe that the first step is to acknowledge the place you are in. Look back and start to understand and accept your past, your family patterns, conditioning, and beliefs. Look at your present, the challenges you face and the opportunities you have. You will then feel empowered to look forward to the future with hope.

It's important to understand that ADHD will affect us all uniquely, at different times, and to remember to be gentle with yourself. On the opposite page are some thoughts on how you may be able to make daily life easier right now.

Strategies to take forward

- Take time to recognise the challenges your ADHD causes you day-to-day, and allow yourself more space and time as you need it.
- Remember that it's okay to have some bad days. Be kind to yourself and focus on establishing wellbeing practices that you can turn to when times are tough.
- Trust the adaptive strategies you've already instinctively created to help you manage life. If running, having an assistant, weight training, drinking caffeine, or paying for a cleaner have helped you without any ill effects, keep doing them and salute the guidance of your inner wisdom.
- Take time to celebrate the aspects of ADHD that bring you joy, so you can create a positive self-identity and lean into your (many!) strengths.

REFLECTIVE MOMENT

Take time to write a few short affirmations with your particular challenges and joys of ADHD in mind. These can be brief statements that summarise how you feel about your ADHD – perhaps laying to rest some ghosts from your past, accepting yourself, or setting down hopes for the future. You can turn back to this when you need some extra support and TLC. You are your own greatest advocate. Here are some examples to get the creative juices flowing:

'I feel compassion for myself and the challenges I have faced.'

'I'm deserving and worthy of love, care, support, and understanding.'

'I have the resilience and power to create a happy and balanced life for myself.'

CHAPTER 2

Soothe Your Anxiety

On our journey towards embracing a happier and more fulfilled life with ADHD, acknowledging our anxiety and working out manageable ways to lessen the mental load is vital. Here, we'll explore why anxiety can be such a challenge for ADHD women and how we can go about calming and soothing it.

THE PROBLEM

Living with heightened anxiety

Not being able to switch off your incessant thoughts can be one of the biggest challenges of living with ADHD. As you've chosen to read this book, it's likely you can relate to a lifetime of having an overactive mind.

Sometimes this is incredibly useful, enabling us to become more resourceful and imaginative, but it's more often exhausting and depleting. In fact, one of my husband's favourite quips since meeting me over 23 years ago, is: 'I'd hate to live inside your head'. Helpful? No. Validating? Yes.

Anxiety has always been a part of my life, and yet I've only recently learnt to recognise it. While I have brilliantly fast-paced ideas, my brain also presses fast-forward on situations in a way that can lead me into a spiral of terrifying fears. This is one of the double-edged swords of ADHD, and it's not just my experience but something I hear about from most of my ADHD clients. It can play out in both externalised and internalised presentations. I see anxiety and ADHD as toxic best friends, both tend to make each other a little worse. So, how can we learn to dial down our anxiety in order to dial up our happiness?

INWARD & OUTWARD PRESENTATIONS

An internalised presentation means behaviours are directed inward;[5] you are likely to feel highly anxious and may want to withdraw from other people. An externalised presentation is more likely to lead to outward-facing behaviours such as impulsivity, physical restlessness, extreme fatigue, productivity paralysis, over-reactivity, frequent rages, lack of patience, irritability, and verbal and physical expressions of anger.

BREAKING IT DOWN

The cycle of anxiety

One of the most excruciating things about anxiety is that it builds: anxiety breeds anxiety. But with increased awareness and compassion, and noticing what is at the root of our anxious thoughts, we're better equipped to press pause and work *with* and no longer against them.

Many of us experience increased anxiety when overwhelmed by the pressures and expectations of life. In these situations, we might think that staying in control and managing everything ourselves will help prevent the things we're anxious about from happening. That as long as things are done our way, and there's no change to the plans we've meticulously carved out, then everything will be okay. However, this rigid thinking only creates more anxiety, and can leave us in a constant state of stress and fear. Our bodies can respond by becoming inflamed, mirroring our internal chaos with pain, autoimmune issues, migraines, gut problems, and more.[6] It's a vicious cycle.

As bleak as this might sound, the reason why I'm painting this picture is so you can learn to recognise your own cycles of anxiety; this awareness will help you to feel more empowered. Life is always going to throw challenges at us, and as with everything, we have to take the rough with the smooth and know there will be ebbs and flows. How we react to these bumps is down to us.

REFLECTIVE MOMENT

Take some time to think about all the significant areas of your life that make you anxious. Can you make a list of the first few that spring to mind? Be honest and list even the smallest things.

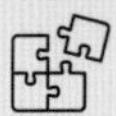

The default mode network

There are many moments of realisation after we become aware of our ADHD, and some are so jaw-dropping that we can't believe we've gone through most of our adult lives without having received the memo. For me, this shock came when I spoke to an ADHD doctor and expert, Dr Ned Hallowell; he explained to me about new neuroscientific evidence connecting ADHD, rumination, and anxiety to a part of our brain called the Default Mode Network (DMN).

New research points to people with ADHD being skewed towards having a more active DMN and finding it more challenging to activate the Task Positive Network (TPN).[7] Although this sounds like a negative trait, when we are aware of our brain's wiring, we can do something about it. Our brain is plastic and can evolve and change according to how we choose to train it. This is why our thoughts, words, and beliefs matter.

Once I understood this vital element of the ADHD brain, it helped me remove some of the blame I put on myself. It allowed me to distance myself from the belief that I should instinctively be able to control myself, and I now know that this is a skill I have to work on. I have had to learn tools and techniques to ground and calm myself in order to relax my amygdala (the part of the brain that keeps watch for danger and controls emotions) and regulate the stress hormone cortisol in my body.

WHAT IS THE DMN?

This is the part of our brain responsible for negative repetitive thinking (known medically as maladaptive ruminative thinking), and studies show that people with ADHD tend to have a more active DMN.[8] The opposing network that works alongside the DMN is the TPN, neural pathways linked to creativity and imagination. To activate the TPN, engage in self-compassion, rest, mindfulness, and awareness of the senses.

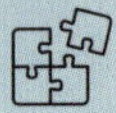

Controlling the DMN

DR NED HALLOWELL, board-certified psychiatrist and world authority on adhd

> *Our greatest gift, as people with ADHD, is our imagination. But it's also our worst enemy. And that's because of the DMN. When your imagination is engaged and you're starting something new, four different regions of the brain light up, and together that's called the TPN. That's when you're at your best. But when the task is complete, the TPN shuts down, and what lights up instead are four other regions of the brain: still your imagination, but another part of it that's called the DMN.*
>
> *Everyone with ADHD has got to know about the DMN, which I call 'the demon' because it sends out negative messages, telling you that you haven't done enough and don't deserve success. It makes you bash yourself in horrible ways. And the reason you keep feeding the demon with your attention is because your ADHD brain is always looking for stimulation. Contentment is too bland. People don't say, 'she was riveted in contentment', but they do say, 'she was riveted in self-hatred and despair and fear and worry.'*
>
> *The DMN is absolutely gripping – it's horrible, but it's gripping. When it takes hold, you go into a kind of stupor of brooding and ruminating, and you just sit there staring at the wall or at the window or wherever. The message that you've got to take in couldn't be simpler, but it's hard to enact: you need to redirect your attention. It's like not looking at the accident on the side of the road: you've got to look the other way – and the minute you do that, the DMN shuts down. It can't survive without your attention. But we tend to feed the demon, because it's stimulating.*
>
> *This is one of the most powerful lessons learned in the past few years: how our great gift, our imagination, can turn into the DMN: a terrible enemy. The positive is that you can control it – not with medication, but by redirecting your attention.*

SCAFFOLDING TO BUILD YOU UP

Identifying anxious thoughts

Let's look at specific ways that anxiety can present so we can identify and manage it when it appears. Remember, there may be many layers of anxiety that will need peeling away. We can't expect to rid ourselves of it completely, but we can lessen the load incrementally each day.

Anxiety and the inner critic

You may not even know that anxiety plays out as a fixating and catastrophising voice in your head. It's important to recognise it: it's the internal narrative that questions or belittles everything you do, and in turn causes anxiety to mount. It may have been with you since childhood, solidified by ongoing criticism from parents, teachers, or toxic friendships. It presents as your true and authentic self, but it focuses on criticising and undermining you and your efforts.

Here's how it can sound: '*You can't; you shouldn't; you have to; don't embarrass yourself; you're broken; you're not good enough.*' You may notice that this voice sometimes translates into certain behaviours that you may feel ashamed of, from struggling to be organised to emotional dysregulation.

IN HER SHOES

I was a huge overthinker and analysed every situation and every word. I always felt anxious and could never understand why others handled life so much better than me. Eventually, I was diagnosed with anxiety and depression and medicated for this.

Claire 43

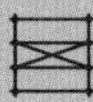

There may be some cases where we have to do extra work, but equally there will be times when we can stand in our power and know that we are worthy.

Speak to your inner critic

When you begin the work of noticing and creating awareness of your inner critic, you have to go slow and be compassionate, especially if there has been trauma from your past that has been feeding into this voice. Thinking of your inner critic as something external (not the 'real you') can be a helpful way to take control of it. You might even like to give it a name and talk or write to it directly. Here's an example of how I speak to my inner critic (let's call her Jen).

> **Hello Jen,**
> *You've always been part of me. Thank you for being there when I thought I needed you to keep me safe. At times, your criticism has stopped me from doing impulsive things. But more often than you have helped me, you have made me feel not good enough and less capable than other people. You've held me back, and now I'm curious about accepting myself and growing. You can rest now and allow me to be led by the voices of kindness and truth.*
> **Kate**

Our inner critic is unique to each of us, often stemming from childhood limiting beliefs, and it won't disappear easily. When it realises it's at risk, its ego will take a hit and it will have a diva strop many, many times over – we just need to keep reinforcing that it is no longer fit for purpose, using our newfound awareness of our ADHD wiring.

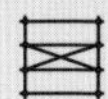

Anxiety and imposter syndrome

'Imposter syndrome' is a phrase we often hear, especially in female communities, and it can be another key source of anxiety. It's incredibly common in those with ADHD. No matter how many accomplishments we have, it means thinking we must have cheated the system in some way and don't deserve to be where we are.

Part of the reason this resonates so strongly with the ADHD community is that we have often had a more difficult path, particularly to academic or professional success. It's quite common that we will have had to work harder, overcompensating for our organisation, executive functioning, working memory, or processing differences. Given the way that ADHD presents, it's likely we'll have internalised societal messages from teachers and managers that we're lazy, not trying hard enough, dysfunctional, and doing things wrong – all of which provide fertile ground for the idea that we don't deserve to be where we are now.

IN HER SHOES

I always felt like there was something wrong with me because I wasn't like other mothers: I was never organised, my house was clean but never tidy; I yelled too much at my children. I honestly felt like a failure. My kids have ADHD, and I have long suspected I have it myself. The thought that 'I am just useless' holds me back from being tested and fully accepting that it might be ADHD.

Kelly, 42

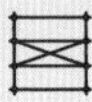

Challenge your imposter syndrome by asking yourself the following questions:

- Think about what you've achieved or excelled at in life: what do you know to be authentic about it?
- What hard evidence do you have that you are suitable for the job/career/education you're currently in or want to do? Do you have testimonials, a degree, or positive feedback? Or is there something you're personally proud of and know you're brilliant at? Keep this in a special 'hype file' so that when you're feeling sensitive to rejection or your self-esteem is low, you can refer back to it. Put it on your desktop or in a physical box that's easy to find when you need a self-worth boost.
- What doubts do you have? For example: 'everyone seems to know more than me', 'I can't do the accounts', or 'I'm not educated enough'. Let it all out, purge all the negative thoughts, and then challenge them. It's okay to have wobbly days, and, as women, we are contending with daily hormonal and ADHD mood swings. This is a *lot* to navigate.
- What is truly important to you? Is it connection with family, love, nature, health, or a feeling of safety? We sometimes need to gain perspective and step out of our ever-running, self-critical thoughts. I find that when I focus on the bigger picture and ask myself what really matters, the worries I'm hyperfocusing on become pretty insignificant.
- Why are you worthy of being where you are or where you want to be? I love asking this question because we all have such unique gifts that are desperately trying to break out.

Recognise your gifts

Every person on this planet has something weird and wonderful to offer. It's so easy to compare, and to live our lives wishing we were doing things like others or that we had what they have, but when we break it down, we know that what *they're* doing wouldn't feel authentic to *us*.

It's crucial to take some time to recognise what our gifts are, and seeing how they have been delivered in a way that is tailored to us can help us to overcome imposter syndrome. It allows us to recognise the purpose we bring to the world. There is space for us all to realise our gifts, but first we must believe in ourselves.

Sometimes, we must break down our stories and beliefs to access the truth, and then work on our self-compassion.

REFLECTIVE MOMENT

When you're ready, look back at your list of things that made you anxious from the start of the chapter. Can any of them be traced back to your inner critic or imposter syndrome?

TOOLS TO HELP

Calm anxiety

We're going to look at some specific tools and techniques to quell anxiety – calming the part of the brain that controls emotions, helping our brain to think in different ways, and allowing us to activate the TPN as needed.

Grounding breath technique

This is an effective technique to manage anxiety if you're in public. It focuses on engaging the senses and anchoring the mind to the present moment, interrupting the cycle of anxious thoughts and sensations.

1. First make yourself comfortable. If you're sitting, try to keep your back straight and feet flat on the ground. Allow your hands to rest gently on your lap or by your sides.
2. Now it's time to focus on your senses. Begin by taking a few gentle breaths, then follow the simple steps opposite to bring you mindfully into your present moment.
3. Take some deep, slow breaths, noticing how your senses are fully activated. Try inhaling through your nose, allowing your stomach to expand, then exhaling slowly through your mouth. With each breath, imagine sending roots down from your body into the ground, anchoring you firmly in the present.
4. Stick with the deep breathing for several minutes, focusing on all your senses, until you feel your anxiety begin to lessen. Each time your mind wanders to anxious thoughts, gently bring it back to your senses and your breath.

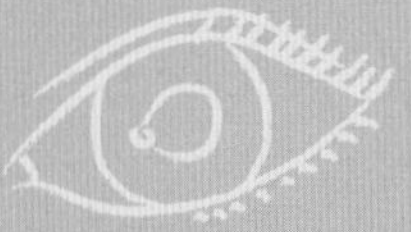

Choose **FIVE** things you can **SEE** around you. Try to pick out small details you may usually overlook. Take time to truly see these things and concentrate on them.

Notice **FOUR** things you can **TOUCH OR FEEL**. Perhaps this is the texture of your clothing, the surface you're sitting on, or the air on your skin.

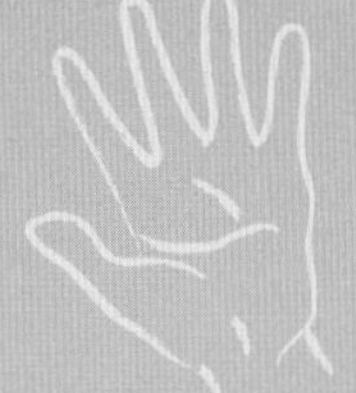

Listen for **THREE** things you can **HEAR**. Notice the sounds in your environment, both near and far. Be aware of how the sounds ebb and flow.

Identify **TWO** things you can **SMELL**. Are there cooking aromas wafting past, or the smell of flowers or perfume? If you can't immediately smell anything, try to recall two scents you have enjoyed in the past.

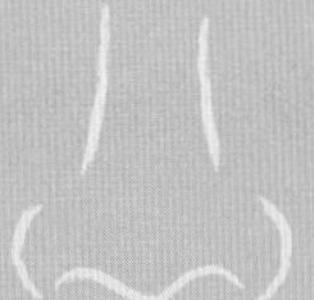

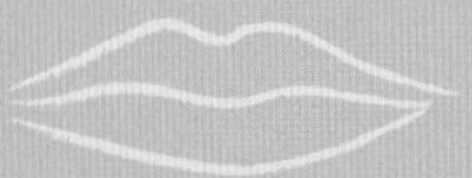

Identify **ONE** thing you can **TASTE**. Focus on the current taste in your mouth, or imagine a taste you find comforting or pleasurable.

Emotional Freedom Technique (EFT): tapping

Cortisol and adrenaline are hormones that our body releases to help us in times of stress. Cortisol raises blood sugar by releasing glucose into the bloodstream, and adrenaline increases the heart rate – both of which give us energy when we feel under attack.

Tapping helps to reduce cortisol and adrenaline and calms the amygdala. It also helps release suppressed emotions. Even though we're bringing up trauma, tapping on the powerful energetic meridian points simultaneously regulates and calms our bodies and nervous systems so we don't become too overwhelmed.

1. Choose a negative self-belief that speaks strongly to you in this moment. I've chosen a belief that I relate to and hear a lot from my clients: 'I am broken' or 'I feel like a failure'.
2. Rate how strong this belief currently feels from 1–10 (the most extreme). For instance, it feels pretty strong at an 8 right now.
3. What emotions are coming up? Where in your body can you feel them? Can you visualise a colour? I often feel strong negative emotions stuck in my throat or as tension in my shoulders.
4. Start tapping on the side of your hand and use a statement such as, 'Even though I believe I'm a failure, I choose to accept that this is how I feel right now and send myself love and compassion.'
5. Do a second round of tapping on the side of your hand, repeating the belief; finish with, 'And that's okay; I accept that this is how I feel right now and send myself some love.'
6. Do a third round, repeating the belief while tapping on the side of the hand; finish by saying: 'I choose to believe that things can improve.' Refrain from bringing in positive words unless they feel authentic and deeply truthful.
7. After three tapping rounds, take a deep breath and measure from 1–10 how true your belief feels now. Do they feel lighter? Did other thoughts or new perspectives come to the surface?

8 Now tap on the face and body points, each time stating how you're feeling. By tapping on the correct body areas to help stimulate the meridian points (the body's energy pathways) while stating truthful comments, you will feel a release – which might be yawning, crying, or a feeling of the emotion moving through your body. Notice where you're holding on to tension, and tap on uncomfortable sensations such as tightness in your throat, pain in your shoulder, or tension in your neck.

9 As you move through each round of tapping on a meridian point, take a deep breath and measure how true your belief feels now. Has your number gone down?

10 The rational side of the brain will want a logical explanation for why you're feeling lighter or less overwhelmed by worries, but try to let this go and simply be open to the release.

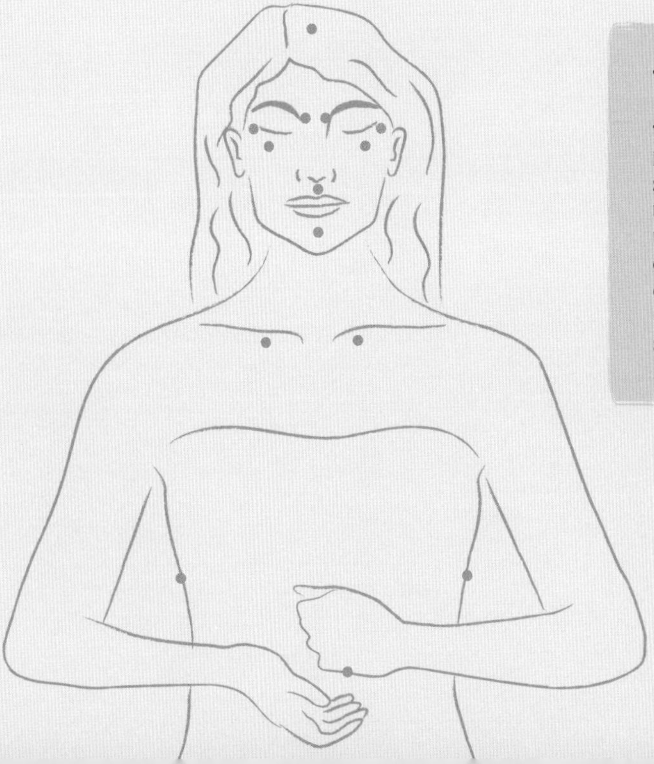

TAPPING POINTS

Top of head
Inner eyebrow
Side of eye
Under eye
Under nose
Chin
Collarbone
Under arm
Side of hand

APBR technique

Another powerful way to self-regulate and feel more grounded when anxiety hits is to focus on breathing intentionally and actively. I call this APBR, which stands for Awareness, Pause, Breathe, and Respond. Let's look at each in turn.

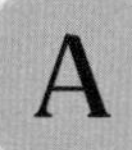

A

AWARENESS

Create awareness around your triggers. Notice what happens in a situation when you lose your temper or feel dysregulated, and how you experience it in your body. Awareness helps us feel more in control and means we can recognise the signs next time.

P

PAUSE

If you can, allow yourself to pause. Give yourself space to recognise what's going on. This provides you with an opportunity to choose how you want to react.

B

BREATHE

Take five long breaths and give yourself this time to choose how you want the situation to develop. Five breaths can make a huge difference to how we can potentially 'turn the ship around'. This is buying you time so that you can choose to...

R

RESPOND

Notice that's R for respond, not react! Responding comes from pausing and breathing, whereas reacting comes straight from our emotions. With this action, we are actively stepping out of the more destructive spotlight of the DMN and intentionally using a 'dimmer switch' to light up the TPN. Think of it like using this gentle dimmer switch to illuminate another area of the room.

Strategies to take forward

Learning to manage your anxiety is one of the biggest game-changers when it comes to living and enjoying life as an adult woman with ADHD. These are the key steps you can take to understand your anxiety and bring it under control.

- Take time to recognise the triggers of when you are feeling anxious, and allow yourself time to notice, pause, and reflect.
- Try to acknowledge and actively externalise your anxious emotions, inner critic, and imposter syndrome – tell yourself gently that they are just thoughts and are not necessarily true.
- Remember to show yourself compassion when things don't work out the way you hoped, and try to intentionally reduce the pressure and expectations you put on yourself.
- Remind yourself that you are more self-aware, resilient, and empowered than you may sometimes think, and always try to speak to yourself with kindness and grace. You deserve it.

REFLECTIVE MOMENT

When you have the time and energy, think about the questions below. They are designed to help you identify the triggers (big and small) that make you anxious. You might like to journal them so you can track your progress.

What normally triggers you to feel anxious or dysregulated?

How do you feel in your body, nervous system, and brain in this situation?

What tools have previously helped calm you or your children in difficult moments?

What new tools have you been inspired to try from this chapter?

CHAPTER 3

Understand Rejection Sensitive Dysphoria

Emotional dysregulation can be one of the more challenging aspects of living with ADHD. For many of us, this is linked to Rejection Sensitive Dysphoria (RSD), a condition causing extreme emotional sensitivity. This chapter looks at how RSD often presents in women with ADHD and how to manage these deeply painful emotions.

THE PROBLEM

Emotional sensitivity and ADHD

RSD can show up in a variety of subtle ways, often intertwined with other symptoms of ADHD. While many people relate to the pain of rejection or feeling left out, the difference for those with RSD is that this becomes debilitating, and the impact is long-lasting.

Understanding and having RSD validated is often a pivotal moment in an ADHD diagnosis. For a professional to explain that it is a verified medical term frequently brings many of us to tears: 'You mean I'm not just overly sensitive and immature?'

Some experts believe that RSD can show up more prominently in women. Societal gender roles can exacerbate RSD symptoms later in life,[9] as well as social conditioning traumas that undiagnosed women and girls may have gone through, such as being ostracised for acting differently and not relating to stereotypical friendship dynamics. When I was growing up, I preferred spending time with my male friends because it felt simpler and easier to navigate than my larger female friendship groups, which often thrived on drama.

WHAT IS RSD?

RSD describes intense emotional pain triggered by extreme feelings of perceived or real rejection or criticism. This might manifest as physical symptoms such as palpitations, migraines, insomnia, back pain, and stomach issues, or feelings of chronic low self-esteem, perfectionism, and avoidance of situations where rejection might occur. It can significantly impact our lives.[10]

BREAKING IT DOWN

Recognising RSD

Let's take a look at what is actually going on in our brains when we experience emotional sensitivity, and how this can affect our daily lives.

The neuroscience of RSD

Advances in neuroimaging have identified brain regions and networks implicated in emotional regulation, social processing, and attention, all of which are relevant to understanding ADHD and RSD.[11] While RSD is primarily characterised by our personal experiences, which may not be directly evident in brain scans, ongoing research in neuroimaging may shed light on the neural mechanisms underlying ADHD, potentially providing insights into the neurobiological basis of RSD. It is helpful for us to understand some key structures of our brilliant brains.

Prefrontal cortex: this area of the brain involves executive functions such as decision-making, impulse control, and emotional regulation. Differing activity in the prefrontal cortex has been observed in those of us diagnosed with ADHD and experts think this may contribute to emotional dysregulation.[12]

Amygdala: one of the oldest and least developed parts of the brain, the amygdala plays a central role in processing emotions, particularly fear and anxiety. Differences in amygdala activation or connectivity have been acknowledged in ADHD brains and may be associated with heightened emotional reactivity.[13]

Fronto-striatal circuitry: connectivity between the prefrontal cortex and subcortical structures like the striatum is crucial for regulating attention and behaviour. Disruptions in this circuitry have been implicated in ADHD and may contribute to difficulties in emotional regulation and response inhibition.[14]

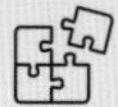

Rejection sensitive dysphoria in ADHD

DR ASAD RAFFI, founder of Sanctum Healthcare, medical director, and lead consultant psychiatrist

" *Understanding the complexity of rejection sensitive dysphoria in ADHD requires a multifaceted approach. The foundational challenges of ADHD stem from executive function deficits: these include issues with planning, organisation, time management, and emotional regulation, leading to functional impairments that prevent individuals with ADHD from reaching their full potential. The achievements they do attain often come at the cost of significant stress and are unsustainable in the long term.*

Ongoing struggles with executive functioning foster a narrative – consciously or subconsciously – where individuals perceive themselves as failures or 'not good enough' and feel a constant sense of under achievement. This negative self-perception is exacerbated by self-doubt, fear of failure, fear of making mistakes, and a significant degree of imposter syndrome.

Self-sabotage frequently follows, compounding the problem. Feedback and criticism from others further reinforces this negative narrative. Research indicates that by age 12, children with ADHD receive 20,000 more negative messages and critiques than neurotypical peers.[15] *This staggering number – over five additional negative comments per day – compounds the internalised belief of inadequacy. A lack of self-belief, stemming from executive functioning deficits and the response of others to this, makes ADHD individuals susceptible to RSD because they do not have a strong foundation from which to manage perceived criticism.*

It's also worth noting that ADHD has a bidirectional relationship with stress and sleep; increased stress and poor sleep can significantly worsen RSD symptoms. "

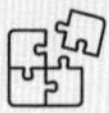

This is the reality of living with RSD, and some of the ways in which it can show up in our daily lives:

- **Hypersensitivity to criticism:** even the mildest criticism will trigger intense emotional reactions, leading to shame and inadequacy.
- **Self-doubt and perfectionism:** you may constantly seek validation from others and not know your own mind. You may feel an intense pressure to excel in various areas of your life to avoid the pain of criticism and rejection.
- **Fear of rejection in relationships:** RSD is often a cause of relationship or friendship issues and can contribute to separation or divorce. Feelings of insecurity can become overpowering and complicated because we don't recognise the root cause (ADHD). We need understanding partners who can show extra compassion and kindness.
- **Overdependence:** you may identify patterns of being overly dependent on your partners (even if they are not right for you) to try to protect yourself from potential hurt.
- **Hypersensitivity to social situations:** maintaining group friendships can feel difficult. We are hyperaware of subtle signs of rejection or disapproval from others, and may read too much into a passing comment or a text and lie awake for nights afterwards wondering what we did or said wrong.
- **Overexplaining:** this is a *big* one for many of us. We tend to over-apologise for perceived mistakes, even when we're not the ones at fault.

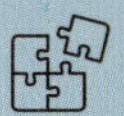

- **Conflict avoidance and people-pleasing:** we may go to great lengths to avoid confrontation, fearing negative reactions from others. As a result, we tend to avoid asserting boundaries and expressing our needs.
- **Imposter syndrome:** we spoke about imposter syndrome in Chapter 2, but it's useful to reflect on it again in this context. Despite obvious evidence of accomplishments, women with imposter syndrome may doubt their abilities and put their successes down to luck or external factors.
- **Physical symptoms:** RSD can manifest as physical symptoms such as tension headaches, palpitations, stomach or gut issues, muscle tension, chronic pain, and insomnia, especially during periods of heightened emotional discomfort.
- **Hormones:** RSD often flares up alongside our menstrual cycle, especially with conditions such as PMDD, and will feel even harder to bear during the last 10–14 days. It may also worsen during puberty, postnatally, and during perimenopause and menopause, thanks to fluctuations in oestrogen impacting our dopamine levels. Fluctuating progesterone levels, which begin to rise just after ovulation, can sometimes have depressive mood-altering influences on neurodivergent women, causing us to become more emotionally sensitive. For more information about hormones, see Chapter 5.

IN HER SHOES

It was only when I suffered a serious episode of RSD with my partner that I realised how much it affected me. I was horrified that it may have possibly ended my relationship. I went to see my GP for an assessment and was diagnosed ADHD.

Julie 58

SCAFFOLDING TO BUILD YOU UP

Settling the mind

The following techniques are things that you can employ to manage RSD and achieve a more settled state of mind.

Psychoeducate yourself

Understanding ADHD and RSD is empowering. Learning about these conditions, their symptoms, and how they manifest can help us become more insightful and less judgemental of our reactions. This allows us to respond with more self-awareness next time a similar trigger comes up.

Therapy and coaching

Seeking out ADHD therapists or coaches who understand RSD may be worth investigating for more specific guidance and support. The power of a professional validating your experience while also offering evidence-based tools can be hugely impactful in emotional healing after an ADHD diagnosis. Neurodivergent-affirming Cognitive Behavioural Therapy (CBT) and Dialectical Behaviour Therapy (DBT) are both beneficial for lessening the impact of RSD.

Therapy, alongside ADHD awareness and understanding, can help us develop new skills for regulating emotions, challenging negative thought patterns, and improving self-esteem. Coaching helps us spot patterns and cycles in our behaviours, thoughts, beliefs, and actions so we're no longer working in our blind spots. Once that happens, we can actively work towards an easier, brighter future loaded with potential.

Self-acceptance and self-compassion

Practising self-compassion involves treating oneself with self-acceptance, forgiveness, kindness, and understanding, especially during difficult moments. This can help counteract the self-critical tendencies often associated with RSD.

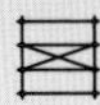

CBT & DBT

CBT focuses on identifying and changing negative thought patterns and behaviours. By using CBT techniques tailored for ADHD, we can challenge ruminative thinking, reframe beliefs about our abilities, and break down daunting activities into manageable and less overwhelming tasks. DBT uses calming CBT techniques alongside practical mindfulness strategies; it emphasises emotional regulation, distress tolerance, and interpersonal effectiveness, which can be pivotal in managing RSD symptoms.

Support and setting boundaries

Connecting with understanding friends, family members, or support groups can provide validation and encouragement. Sharing experiences with others who have ADHD or RSD can reduce feelings of isolation and provide practical advice. Setting boundaries in relationships and at work can help prevent situations that trigger RSD.

Medication support

In some cases, medication prescribed for ADHD symptoms may also help alleviate those of RSD. Working closely with a specialised ADHD healthcare professional to find the right medication and dosage is essential. Unfortunately, with ADHD medication it very often takes trial and error and varying titrations (gradually increasing or decreasing the dose) to find that sweet spot. We know that certain medications can help hugely with emotional dysregulation and RSD. Do your research and advocate for yourself when speaking to your doctor. Our ADHD traits and symptoms are so individualised, as are our genes and nervous systems, and we have to find the options that work best for us.

Building our self-esteem can be especially empowering when we feel like we've been emotionally winded time and time again.

Understand the biology

Key to managing RSD is understanding how it connects to physical bodily processes. Your body contains what is known as the Autonomic Nervous System (ANS); this controls all the bodily processes that we need to happen without us thinking about them (such as breathing). The ANS is subdivided into the sympathetic and parasympathetic systems: the sympathetic nervous system triggers our 'fight or flight' response, while the parasympathetic system helps us to calm down and relax. Actively engaging with the parasympathetic system allows us to pause, giving us space to choose how we want to move forward with more perspective and clarity and *not* react in the moment. For more on the nervous system, see Chapter 4.

CALMING THE NERVOUS SYSTEM

The parasympathetic nervous system is colloquially known as the 'rest and digest' system, as it helps our bodies to process food and energy while we're resting. Breathing slowly helps to slow the fight-or-flight sympathetic nervous system response by telling the body it's time to activate the rest-and-digest parasympathetic system instead. When we breathe slowly, we are telling our bodies that the threat is over and it's time to reduce the cortisol and send blood to our gut to help with digestion, reducing the physical signs of tension and engaging the parasympathetic nervous system.[16]

TOOLS TO HELP

Regulate emotions

Now we'll dive into some tailored strategies to help you to self-regulate your emotional reactivity.

Challenging our RSD

Cognitive restructuring is a helpful CBT technique that helps us challenge unhelpful thoughts triggered by RSD. This simple, flexible method enables us to identify and question negative thoughts and replace them with kinder, more constructive alternatives. For example, if we think, 'Everyone is always with their friends and I'm left out,' we can reframe that thought by reminding ourselves that we often don't enjoy busy social gatherings and would rather see friends in smaller groups.

CATCH
Learn to spot RSD when it's happening. Identify any physical sensations you feel, such as a racing heart. Pause to create some distance, especially if you're still feeling reactive.

↓

CHALLENGE
Get curious about how true these thoughts are. Do you know the whole story? Have you jumped to conclusions or defaulted to 'all or nothing' thinking?

↓

CHANGE
Create a more balanced perspective, such as 'I enjoy seeing my friends in smaller groups' or 'It's okay that I'm not in a noisy restaurant with people I don't feel comfortable with'.

Gently expose yourself to potentially triggering situations

Also known as 'exposure therapy', this may sound drastic, but it simply involves consciously exposing yourself to situations that might trigger RSD in a way that feels controllable to you. This helps safely build tolerance and reduce sensitivity over time.

Take social anxiety, which often goes hand in hand with RSD, as an example. Think about what the worst possible outcome could be in a social situation: for instance, organising a get-together where you fear that no one will come. Now expose yourself to this fear in a way you feel comfortable with. This doesn't have to mean organising huge events; simply inviting a friend you enjoy spending time with to dinner is a good place to start.

Distress tolerance

Learn techniques to cope with frustration and stress without resorting to impulsive actions. Experts in DBT recommend using 'distress tolerance' techniques like 'TIPP' to quickly reduce the intensity of emotional responses when feeling overwhelmed.

T — **TEMPERATURE**
Splash your face with cold water or take an ice bath.

I — **INTENSE EXERCISE**
Try going for a power walk, run, or resistance-based workout.

P — **PACED BREATHING**
Practise techniques such as box breathing (see p.60).

P — **PROGRESSIVE RELAXATION**
Clench and release different muscle groups to reduce tension.

Create a RSD thought journal

When you next experience RSD, take a moment to jot down what's happened, how you interpreted and processed the situation, and what your inner wisdom is telling you. You can record this in a notebook or, if it's more convenient, use the Notes app on your phone. Many of us with ADHD find that externalising our thoughts is a helpful way to process and understand hurtful situations.

AN EXAMPLE FOR YOUR RSD THOUGHT JOURNAL COULD BE

The facts: My boss has asked me for a meeting next week.

My thought: They're not happy with my work and I'm going to be fired.

Evidence for: I have taken some days off sick recently and feel quite burnt out.

Evidence against: They were kind about me having some time off and regularly tell me I'm an asset to the business.

Alternative explanation: They may need to discuss a new project, offer help or accommodations, ask how I'm doing, or offer a different position. It doesn't have to be negative.

Inner wisdom: Perhaps what will come from this is something for the greater good and maybe I can trust that whatever comes from this meeting will be positive.

Calming breathwork

Intentional breathing – 'breathwork' – is a practical and cost-free way to engage the parasympathetic nervous system, calm the mind, ground the body, and manage reactive emotions.

Box breathing (square breathing)

Box breathing is a powerful yet simple relaxation technique that aims to return breathing to its normal rhythm. It's also a great one to use when feeling triggered by RSD, when you are in stressful situations, or for simply helping to refocus the mind.

1. Sit upright in a comfortable chair with your feet flat on the ground.
2. Close your eyes and take a few deep breaths to begin.
3. Inhale through your nose while counting to four slowly. Feel the air enter your lungs.
4. Hold your breath while counting slowly to four. Try not to clamp your mouth or nose shut – simply avoid inhaling or exhaling for four seconds.
5. Begin to exhale for four seconds slowly.
6. Repeat steps 3–5 for four minutes or until calm and focused.

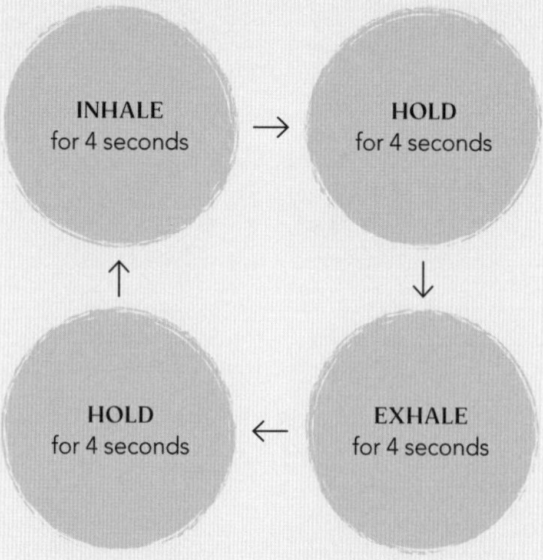

Diaphragmatic breathing (belly breathing)

This technique encourages full oxygen exchange and is a great way to reduce stress.

1 Sit comfortably or lie down, placing one hand on your belly and the other on your chest.

2 Breathe in slowly through your nose, allowing your belly to push your hand out while your chest remains relatively still.

3 Exhale slowly through your mouth or nose, whichever feels more comfortable, engaging your abdominal muscles to help push air out.

4 Repeat this breathing pattern for a few minutes, focusing on the rise and fall of your belly.

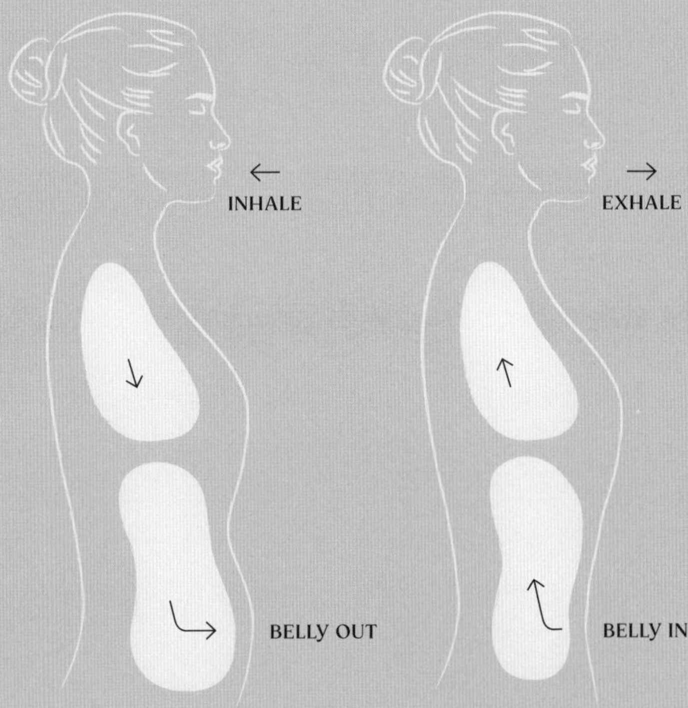

Learn to recognise RSD

Noticing and recognising RSD is half the battle to lessening its impact, and I find this approach helpful for managing and then moving through RSD emotions.

1. ***Be aware***

   First, notice the signs from your body when you are experiencing RSD. Does a feeling form in your throat or the pit of your stomach? Is your heart racing, or your head pounding?

2. ***Don't judge***

   Now, identify your RSD without judgement. Just be aware that it is happening. By naming and recognising RSD, we're taming it. It's no longer a defective character flaw or a weakness; it's simply a tricky component of our ADHD.

3. ***Show self-compassion***

   The key is to speak to the RSD part of us and say something along the lines of: 'I understand that I'm going to have some intense feelings based on this triggering situation. Even though everything feels heightened in my body and emotions, I'm also aware of my tendency towards RSD, and I'm giving myself grace and forgiveness for how I'm reacting right now.'

4. ***Record the feeling***

   Take some time to sit with what you're feeling and write it down. Where in your body can you feel the emotions? Remember to speak to yourself with compassion and kindness as you gently move through your emotions.

Strategies to take forward

- Look out for your specific RSD triggers; note them down to help yourself to feel prepared in future. If you can sense RSD coming before you spiral, you can gain perspective and move out of the situation.
- Practise techniques such as simple breathwork or tapping. Try these when you're calm and settled so they come to you more easily when you need them.
- Develop calming coping mechanisms and healthy distractions. Going for a run or a power walk can help shift negative energy and boost feelgood chemicals in your brain.
- Uphold healthy boundaries. Becoming more assertive with your needs, and noticing any people-pleasing tendencies will allow you to remember that your emotions also matter.
- Practise self-acceptance and self-compassion; it is critical to remember that you are simply a human who sometimes experiences life intensely.
- Accept failures and celebrate achievements. Recognise that we all make mistakes and things often don't go the way we'd hoped.

REFLECTIVE MOMENT

If now feels like a good time, consider the questions below. You might like to journal them, so you can track your progress.

What do you notice in your body when emotional sensitivity or RSD is beginning to flare up?

What coping mechanisms do you already have in place that you know help you?

Can you think of three tools to reach for when your heightened emotions or RSD feel difficult to manage?

CHAPTER 4

Regulate Your Nervous System

This chapter looks at how our nervous systems can become overactive and dysregulated. We'll explore what this feels like, why it's happening, and what we can do to help maintain equilibrium. We'll also look at different ways to self-regulate so we can access our unique coping methods when life feels challenging and overwhelming.

THE PROBLEM

Living with a dysregulated nervous system

If you're reading this book, especially as a late-identified ADHD woman, chances are that the experience of living with a dysregulated nervous system will be nothing new, even if you haven't been consciously aware of it. It is time to address that, to take back control of our overwhelmed brains and exhausted bodies, and to heal.

Long before I knew about my own ADHD, I recognised my overactive nervous system in periods of chronic stress, making me feel wired and jittery – the opposite of how I feel after an hour's yoga or walking in nature. Most neurodivergent people have sensitive nervous systems that crave quiet rest, relaxing restoration, and gentle grounding. However, our ADHD traits can make achieving this sense of calm difficult.

We often have exceedingly high expectations of ourselves and always want to go the extra mile, driven by our need for dopamine. In addition to our compromised executive functioning and working memory challenges, it can seem as though we go round in circles – busy but feeling like we're not achieving much, which causes us to push to keep working and achieving despite being exhausted. It's no wonder our nervous systems are struggling.

IN HER SHOES

Before I understood my ADHD I suffered from serious physical and mental health problems – I felt terrified of everything. With hindsight I began to realise just how dysregulated my nervous system was.

Emma 53

Recognising the symptoms

A dysregulated ADHD nervous system can show up in any of the following ways, all of which we'll investigate in more detail throughout this chapter.

- Overworking, needing to be constantly productive or busy
- Restlessness, or a fear of resting, and an inability to relax, believing that there is always more to do, and we are constantly behind or failing
- Lack of boundaries and engaging in people-pleasing behaviour
- Heightened sensitivity to others' behaviour, or RSD
- Feeling paralysed, with an inability to be productive or initiate tasks
- Experiencing shutdown (a 'freeze' response), overwhelm, and numb detachment
- Adrenal fatigue and burnout

NERVOUS SYSTEM'S FUNCTION

The nervous system is responsible for carrying messages back and forth between the brain and the body. Ideally, this system works like a well-oiled machine, scanning and interpreting what's happening around us and only hitting the panic button if we're under immediate threat. However, when the nervous system is dysregulated and hypervigilant, we often react to perceived threats in a disproportionate way. This might be an overreaction, manifesting as outbursts and anger, or an underreaction like withdrawal or shutting down.

Understanding the cause

We are still in the early stages of understanding the scientific connection between ADHD and our nervous systems. However, through conversations with the ADHD community and on my podcast, I hear about the ADHD lived experience of having a hypervigilant nervous system all the time. These discussions, along with my own research, have led me to believe that this dysregulation often stems from decades-old trauma and challenging life experiences,[17] creating brain/body inflammation. This might include adverse childhood experiences, family dysfunction, addiction, disordered eating, misunderstood health challenges, academic and social rejection, and more. Our nervous systems try to protect us from these unfavourable experiences by acting as an overactive warning operative, alerting us to potential future threats.

Beginning to heal

Unfortunately, trauma is a common component of undiagnosed ADHD, and we must never underestimate the impact of pain we have held on to, struggles we've stayed quiet about, and all the times we've been completely overwhelmed. As you begin your healing journey towards thriving as a neurodivergent woman, taking some time to understand your nervous system and how it affects your health and wellbeing will help you on your way.

I wish there was more information out there about the neurodivergent nervous system, but like many areas of ADHD research, it is still sparse. Instead, you'll have to come with me while I explore what I know to be true for myself and for the many women I have spoken to over the years. We have found validation through the process of connecting lifelong health complications and other struggles to a severely dysregulated and heightened nervous system.

BREAKING IT DOWN

Understanding the nervous system

Let's delve deeper into the complex topic of the nervous system, and explore in more detail the crucial relationship it has with ADHD. By understanding more about how our nervous system works, we can get to a place where we are better able to calm and regulate ourselves.

Fight or flight

If you are living with ADHD, you will probably be familiar with the feeling of 'fight or flight'. The fight-or-flight response is triggered by the sympathetic nervous system to protect you from potentially threatening situations. It might feel like a state of high alert, and can cause a number of physiological changes in preparation for imminent danger, including increased heart rate, improved muscle strength, heightened sensory input, and overactive mental activity.

This response was particularly useful when we were living in caves and needed to keep watch for dangerous animals or threatening enemies; it is perhaps not so helpful when it's triggered by day-to-day experiences such as a negative comment in an email, trolling on social media, or feeling rejected in a social situation. Despite these scenarios not being life-threatening, they trigger our finely-tuned nervous systems to activate the fight-or-flight response.

IN HER SHOES

At my worst, I felt overwhelmed all of the time, crying at work then at home. I would have panic attacks and go into functional freeze where I wasn't able to think straight, or even put sentences together. Eventually my nervous system collapsed and I was unable to function for months.

Sarah 52

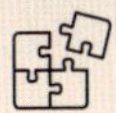

Hypervigilance

Hypervigilance occurs when our fight-or-flight response becomes overactive, leaving us in a persistent state of anxiety. Many of us will have felt this over the years, because several ADHD traits can leave us feeling stuck, unsafe, and disconnected from others.

Take our relationship with time, for example. Differences in time perception means that we can often overestimate or underestimate how long something may take. This leads us to be chronically late in a way that feels beyond our control, creating huge amounts of anxiety and dread, which weighs heavily on our nervous systems.

Another example is the procrastination/perfectionism combination. We often struggle to initiate a project unless we have either done a PhD in the subject or spent a whole day hyperfixating on every intricate detail. It can also mean not starting anything unless we know the deadline is looming so close that we have no other choice than to stay up all night guzzling energy drinks and writing the 10,000-word dissertation that is due by 9am. After this, it may take our cortisol and adrenal levels a week to recover, and we might experience burnout. And that, my friends, is what I call putting our nervous systems into a heightened, frenzied state.

REFLECTIVE MOMENT

Take a few minutes to read back over the examples above: do any of these experiences resonate with you? You might like to note down some of the times when you've experienced something similar, and how this made you feel.

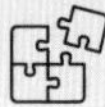

The polyvagal theory

Devised by Dr Stephen Porges, the polyvagal theory is based on the belief that there's a strong link between our nervous system's subconscious physiological responses (such as breathing and heartbeat) and our emotions and behaviours. In particular, it homes in on how we respond to danger in our environment, and how our body subconsciously reacts to it. Learning about the polyvagal theory is particularly useful for those of us who are highly sensitive to stress. By understanding our physiological state, polyvagal theory argues that we can understand our emotional responses, too.

Dr Porges developed his initial concept of the polyvagal theory to include what he called a 'polyvagal ladder metaphor', using an image of a ladder (see p.85) to describe how humans respond to stress.

- **Top rung (ventral vagal):** a safe, connected, and social state. We feel in flow, energised, passionate, and hopeful. We are open to social engagement.
- **Middle rung (sympathetic):** a mobilised fight-or-flight state. We feel reactive, anxious, impatient, agitated, angry, or hypervigilant. We are ready to spring into action and escape the perceived danger.
- **Bottom rung (dorsal):** a collapsed, shutdown state. We feel numb, burnt out, and unable to communicate and regulate our emotions. We may struggle to get out of bed or ask for help. We feel helpless, lacking in hope or solutions. In this state, we sense extreme danger and become immobilised.

Porges observed that we move through these states sequentially in response to external and internal stimuli, and that the movement can be fluid and rapid. The ideal state for a human to live in is the ventral state, yet for many of us this is sadly too fleeting, and we find ourselves more often navigating the sympathetic and dorsal states.

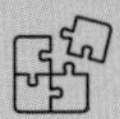

Taking time to notice where we are in our bodies allows us to respond with more clarity and groundedness.

Your home-from-home state

As we get to know ourselves, it becomes easier to recognise our 'home-from-home' state, or what is commonly considered our default state of being. Home-from-home states may not always be particularly pleasant or wanted: for example, if you've experienced trauma, you are likely to find yourself stuck in the dorsal state. For many years my home-from-home state was 'fight, flight, or freeze', which is a response activated by the sympathetic nervous system. I was permanently trapped on the middle rung, with my body never able to fully relax.

If you are also set to fight, flight, or freeze mode, there could be many reasons for that: you may have experienced childhood trauma, such as having an abusive family member and needing (quite rightly) to be on guard for self-preservation; or perhaps there has been addiction in your family, where you've had to be alert to what version of a person will show up each day; or it may simply be a consequence of ADHD itself, especially if you've spent many years trying to navigate life undiagnosed. Be gentle with yourself as you learn the states that your body automatically defaults to: these are based on your wider experiences and aren't something that you can easily control.

REFLECTIVE MOMENT

Take some time to reflect on your 'home-from-home' state. Where does it fall on the polyvagal ladder? Note down how your life experiences so far may have contributed to this.

SCAFFOLDING TO BUILD YOU UP

Calming your nervous system

Now it's time to look at simple tweaks you can make to your everyday life to soothe your dysregulated nervous system.

Identify your triggers and glimmers

The author and polyvagal expert Deb Dana builds on Dr Porges' theory (see p.72) by calling traumatic or difficult events that cause us to move down the polyvagal ladder 'triggers' and uplifting, calming, or connecting moments that help us move up 'glimmers'. Learning our triggers and glimmers can be helpful as we establish ways to regulate our nervous systems.

We may already be adept at identifying the triggers that cause us to feel disconnected, dysregulated, fearful, or anxious. For instance, you might have very specific memories from childhood of being excluded or not fitting in, so being in a situation similar to this as an adult can be triggering.

Homing in on our glimmers can take a bit more practice because of the strong negativity bias we possess as humans. Think back to a time where you felt safe and connected; perhaps it was on your own, with a friend, or with a loved one. Glimmers can feel different and unique to everyone, but you'll likely notice feeling warm, tranquil, connected, secure, and grounded. By taking some deep breaths, closing our eyes, and recalling our easily accessible glimmers, we can move from an immobilised dorsal vagal state through to a sympathetic mobilised state, and towards a connected ventral vagal state. The more we practise this, the more empowered and in control we feel, knowing that external situations don't have to derail us.

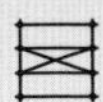

Switch off

Scrolling on our phones for hours on end can activate our fight, flight, or freeze mode, especially in the morning, and makes us feel more hypervigilant. Becoming more intentional with technology and marking-out time to really switch off is crucial.

Our neurodivergent brains are wired for dopamine seeking, meaning we can have more addictive tendencies than neurotypical people. Some of this dopamine-seeking behaviour is also used as a way to self-regulate, and is often called 'stimming' (short for self-stimulating behaviour). Stimming, for neurodivergent people, is a calming way to rest, regulate, or recharge, which is why you may see ADHD children with chewed sleeves, bitten nails, or picked cuticles, doodling or wanting to use fidget toys. As adults this needn't be shamed, we just have to find the best sensory output for us.

It's a never-ending paradox that will continue to try to trip us up unless we create awareness and understanding – which is not so easy when we're in the thick of it. To make their devices as addictive as possible, technology companies like to trigger our sympathetic nervous systems so that we stay hypervigilant and keep checking in with our tech. For this reason, I turn off all my notifications, including news app alerts, to prevent me from falling further into a state of heightened stress and distraction. For those of us living with ADHD, we really must become mindful, especially in the evening and morning, of the technology that we subscribe to in our tech-obsessed always 'on' age, if we are to protect our dopamine-sensitive brains.

A mantra to repeat: the way you do things isn't wrong or broken, it's just different to others. And that's okay.

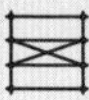

The importance of sleep

A good night's sleep is key to our nervous system's wellbeing; when we are asleep, the level of sympathetic nervous system activation decreases,[18] along with our heart rate and blood pressure, allowing us time to reduce the inflammation in our bodies, settle our brains, and reset. Unfortunately, sleep issues and ADHD are closely related, with our hyperactive brains and bodies (such as the ADHD co-condition known as Restless Leg Syndrome, or RLS) often preventing us from falling asleep or maintaining good-quality sleep. This means our sympathetic nervous system doesn't get the downtime it needs. It is also not uncommon to wake up early in the morning, our eyes pinging open as we remember our endless to-do lists, jolting our nervous systems into a cortisol-induced sympathetic state almost immediately.

Nighttime procrastination

As women, we may relate to the 'revenge nighttime procrastination' pull, when we find an activity to engage us rather than settle to sleep; this is a strategy many busy people use to claw back 'lost' time from their day.[19] Although it feels good at the time, it means the cycle continues and we don't get those quality hours of sleep that help rest our nervous system for yet another manic day ahead.

The impact of lack of sleep on our ADHD symptoms can be debilitating.[20] Apart from feeling physically exhausted and mentally drained after a lousy night's sleep, I think we can all relate to feeling far more irritable, impatient, and lacking in focus. Sleep is a crucial component of our brain's health, and as ADHD is a neurobiological disorder, we rely even more heavily on our brain functioning at its peak to thrive in life. Sleep has an important part to play in helping us organise our memories, it affects our mood, energy, motivation, and executive functioning, and impacts on our learning abilities. It is also vital for the brain, nervous system, and cardiovascular health.[21]

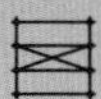

Sleep and hormones

For women with ADHD, our hormones may also have an extreme impact on our sleep, especially during perimenopause and menopause, which is why so many women seek an ADHD assessment around that time. For me, my sleep challenges as I hit perimenopause exacerbated my ADHD traits. Between ovulation and our menstrual period, our oestrogen and progesterone levels drop, which contributes to low mood, anxiety, and insomnia, and lessens our resilience to stress. Hormone Replacement Therapy (HRT) was a true game-changer for me, as the non-synthetic progesterone helped me feel calmer and finally allowed me to achieve a better quality of sleep in the second half of my cycle. As perimenopause continues, finding an optimum level of progesterone is vital to help us sleep better, feel more resilient, calm, emotionally regulated, and empowered.

Sleep is serious business

With ADHD, we must prioritise sleep hygiene to bolster our brains as much as possible, meaning that phones, tablets, and other electronic gadgets need to be hidden away from our dopamine-seeking hands. Ensuring our circadian rhythms are a priority by getting morning sunlight and reducing the artificial lighting as evening draws in is a powerful way to encourage better-quality sleep. I've also found that as I get older, investing in better-quality bedding and pillows has been helpful – I'd now much rather have a fabulous pillow and mattress that I sleep on every day than a designer handbag gathering dust on the shelf. Oh, and another tip: I swear by magnesium glycinate, ear plugs, calming essential oils, opening the window to cool the room, and getting black-out blinds. For me, sleep is serious business because if I'm sleeping okay, then my ADHD symptoms are easier to manage and I feel like a better version of me.

Hydration

When we're dehydrated, our sympathetic nervous system is activated, making us feel more anxious, irritable, and impatient.[22] I can feel the impact of not being properly hydrated on my energy, mood, and concentration almost immediately. Simply put, 75% of our brain mass is water, so when we are dehydrated our brain, which is already working harder than most neurotypical brains, lacks much-needed fuel.

Staying hydrated is scientifically proven to make a difference to our wellbeing. In a study comparing those who have a low daily water intake of below 1.2 litres (2 pints) and those who have a high daily water intake of 2–4 litres (3.5–7 pints), increasing water intake for the low group had a positive impact on sleep patterns, whereas decreasing water intake for those who drank a higher amount negatively affected not only sleep but also mood.[23] This study wasn't focused on ADHD individuals, but knowing our sensitive systems, the effects could be even more magnified. Drink water in whatever way you can, and when you drink it, notice how it's making you feel and whether it helps you cope better during your day.

Remember that caffeine and energy drinks are diuretics, meaning that they actively dehydrate you when you drink them. If caffeine is helpful for your ADHD, ensure you're drinking an extra glass of water alongside your coffee.

ACTIVATE THE VAGUS NERVE

The vagus nerve is part of the larger autonomic nervous system and is a combination of 12 cranial nerves in the parasympathetic nervous system (see p.56). Its responsibilities include calming the body after stressful situations, controlling mood, regulating inflammatory responses, and carrying signals from the brain to other parts of the body. Daily practices such as deep breathing, chanting, cold-water exposure, singing, yoga, and mindfulness can help stimulate the vagus nerve and take you out of a state of fight, flight, or freeze – a powerful way to calm and regulate your body.

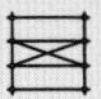

It's time to learn to trust yourself, listen to your body – with all its subtle signs – and learn how it's communicating with you.

Movement

Exercise is crucial, not only to our physical wellbeing but also for our mental health. Exercise boosts the number of blood vessels, stimulating our brain and that all-important vagus nerve.[24] Our bodies are designed to move, and when we don't do that, 'pent-up energy gets stuck inside and creates more stress,' according to Jonathan Hoban, the pioneer of walking therapy and author of *Walk With Your Wolf*. Hoban says, 'I recommend an hour of walking throughout the day – ideally a minimum of two 30-minute walks – to get your brain working at its best. This amount of time helps reduce your cortisol levels and calm down the adrenal glands. Too much of the stress hormone cortisol can cause increased anxiety and adrenal fatigue.'

When navigating a later-in-life ADHD diagnosis, there are often decades' worth of big emotions to dismantle, and releasing these can help us feel optimistic about the present and excited about the future. Somatic exercises, such as tai chi and quigong, are incredibly powerful to help us release 'stuck' past emotions and calm the nervous system. A somatic movement is one that's practised with the intention of focusing on the internal experience of the movement rather than the external appearance or end result. Essentially, we are moving our bodies to explore where we can feel tension and stuck energy.

If you have experienced pain, tension, jaw ache, migraines, or have stuck trauma, working with a specialist somatic experiencing practitioner or somatic movement instructor will help you process emotions through gentle, nonjudgemental movement in your body. You can do somatic exercises at home, but I would recommend working with a professional first, so you know what to do with these emotions once they are released.

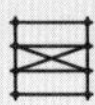

ADHD and the nervous system

ALLEGRA FOXLIE, trauma-informed bodyworker and author of *HTR: Hormone Tension Release*

❝ *Our nervous system is an electrochemical messaging system that governs all physical and emotional health. It includes the brain, spinal cord – which is a major energy highway – and fascia – the sensory connective tissue that surrounds all organs. Think of the body as a massive internet, the nervous system sends signals to our endocrine (hormonal) control centre, which then messages our body's vital organs – ovaries, thyroid, etc. – telling them what hormones to produce at the right time of day, and in what quantities. It also has a controlling influence on our immune system and vasomotor function.*

Trauma and stress are common in individuals with ADHD, often due to a higher likelihood of adverse childhood experiences (ACEs), especially for those who grew up undiagnosed. These experiences can lead to dysregulation of the nervous system, meaning our body might not be getting the right messages and in some instances might not get any messages at all. Meaning our harmonious system – the body – can fail in surprisingly hard to diagnose ways.

The more trauma and stress you have, the more likely you are to suffer from health problems linked to the nervous system, so ADHD women are particularly at risk. This includes period pain, Premenstrual Dysphoric Disorder (PMDD), Premenstrual Exacerbation (PME), fibromyalgia, fibroids, and autoimmune disorders such as complex chronic pain and chronic fatigue. Around 80% of people who suffer from autoimmune disorders are women, and that skyrockets during perimenopause and menopause, when inflammation increases rapidly.

There are a number of things that you can do to support your nervous system. If you have a traumatic past, I recommend working with a trauma-informed therapist. Learning body techniques to calm and regulate the nervous system can be

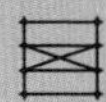

hugely beneficial. Releasing trauma and stress from the body helps the brain to process the past, calming the nervous system and bringing the body and mind back to balance 'homeostasis'.

When you feel dysregulated, simple but effective short-term strategies you can use include:

- **Splash your hands, feet, and face with really cold water.** *This shocks the nervous system, which can be a great temporary solution for anxiety.*

- **Breathwork**. *Try breathing in through the nose, down to the belly for a count of four, then breathe out through the mouth for a count of eight (doubling up on the exhale activates our healing parasympathetic nervous system and slows the heart rate).*

- **Daily physical movement.** *Yoga, Pilates, stretching, jumping, rebounding – all release endorphins, which are calming.*

For deeper long-term change, combining body and talking therapy is recommended. Working with the body first helps to regulate the nervous system, making it easier to focus and take in the talking therapy. Body therapy techniques could include neurogenic tremoring, neurogenic yin, and tension- and trauma-releasing exercises. In these examples, we use involuntary movement to activate the brainstem. This sends an electric charge around the nervous system, rebooting it, regulating it, releasing tension in the fascia, and helping you to process your past.

Deep change within the nervous system is the foundation of emotional happiness. Think of it like building a castle on sand: no matter how great the facade, it is still at risk of sinking. Similiarly, no matter how happy you look on the surface, if your nervous system isn't regulated, you're still likely to collapse. So it's definitely worth putting the time in to learn how to regulate your nervous system and overcome your trauma and stress. ”

TOOLS TO HELP

Soothe your mind and body

We're going to examine some specific strategies to help you manage your nervous system. This practical guidance will help you calm and regulate both your mind and body.

Co-regulation

With co-regulation we can intentionally regulate our emotions and behaviours through supportive interactions with another trusted person.[25]

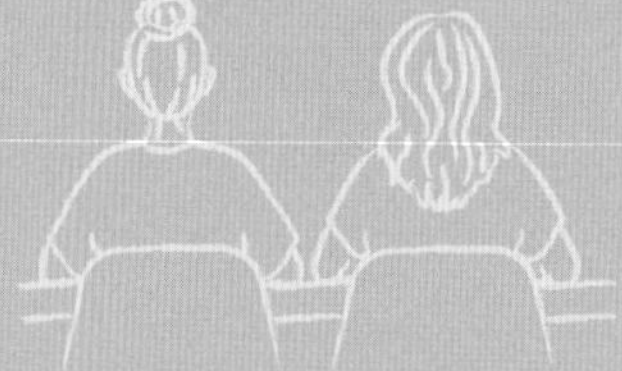

Body doubling: simply sitting next to someone with ADHD to help them complete a task can help prevent paralysing overwhelm.

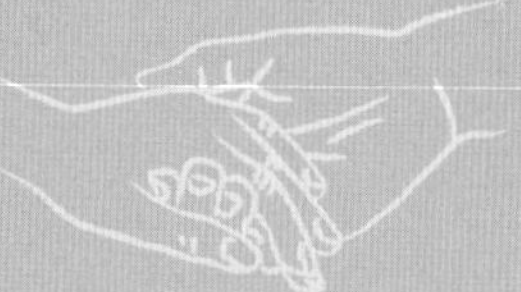

Hand holding: taking someone's hand when they are feeling overwhelmed can help them settle.

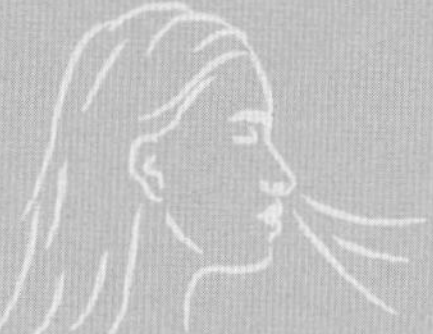

Gentle breathing in tandem: do this for several minutes to help regulate the breath and heart rate and soothe a heightened experience.

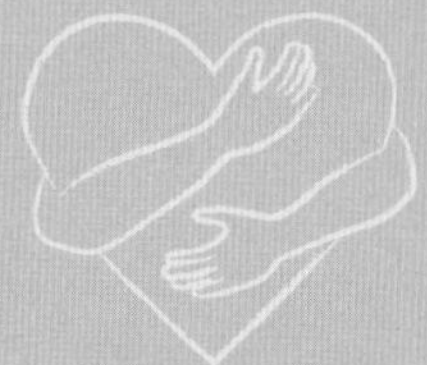

A heart hug: effectively a deep hug where your hearts are both touching. Hold each other until you feel your breathing align and you're able to let out a long exhale.

Understand your window of tolerance

The window of tolerance describes the optimal zone of arousal for feeling adequately regulated and able to function well in daily life. Our nervous systems work effectively in this more regulated state, no longer being thrown off balance by life's challenges. This helps us navigate the inevitable stressors we all face with inner calm, composure, and perspective. Think about what you can do more of to expand your window of tolerance.

HYPERAROUSAL

Hyperarousal is similar to the sympathetic activated state, where we can feel stressed, angry, anxious, and overwhelmed. Symptoms include panic, impulsive behaviour, emotional outbursts, hypervigilance, muscle tightness, and pain.

↓

Things that shrink our window:
stress, trauma, worry, resentment, doomscrolling, being sedentary, lack of boundaries, overcommitting, people-pleasing, lack of sleep, and poor nutrition

↑

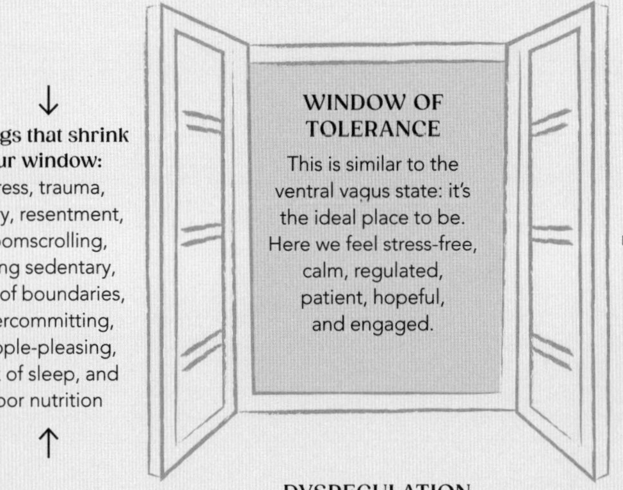

WINDOW OF TOLERANCE
This is similar to the ventral vagus state: it's the ideal place to be. Here we feel stress-free, calm, regulated, patient, hopeful, and engaged.

↑

Things that expand our window:
mindfulness, movement, therapy, sleep, rest, healthy nutrition, hydration, cutting back on alcohol, creativity, time in nature

↓

DYSREGULATION

Dysregulation is similar to the dorsal state. Here, we feel numb, shut down, powerless, disconnected, frozen, and drained. Symptoms include disassociation, numbness, and depression.

Recognising your glimmers and triggers

Earlier in the chapter, we discussed the polyvagal ladder theory (see p.72), which explains how the nervous system moves through a hierarchy of states from safety and connection (ventral vagal) to shutdown (dorsal vagal). The following exercise can help you to identify your unique triggers and glimmers: these are the things that allow you to either move up or down the ladder (see p.74). It will also empower you to recognise your different (and perhaps blended) states and regulate yourself proactively, instead of being subconsciously derailed in daily life without understanding why until it's too late. Take a pen and paper, and answer the questions (opposite) to help you recognise each state and what you can do to move between them.

Glimmers that move me up:
Therapy, expressing anger, crying, somatic movement, yoga, meditation, sleeping well, eating healthily, exercising, spending time with a loved one, switching off social media, having a bath walking the dog, morning sunshine, a day off work, essential oils

Triggers that move me down:
Trauma, PMDD, burnout, anxiety, hormonal upheaval, bad sleep, poor nutrition, stress, feeling misunderstood, experiencing RSD, too much caffeine

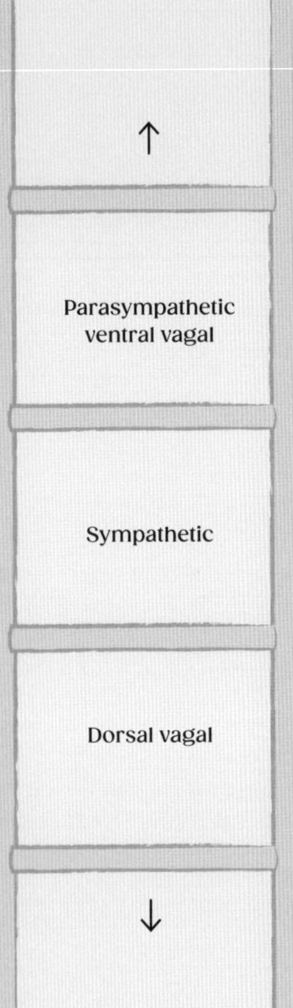

PARASYMPATHETIC VENTRAL VAGAL
Safety, engagement, growth, health, connected, regulated, calm, relaxed

What are your emotions and how does the world feel?

What experiences typically help you find yourself in this state?

What can I do more of to stay in this state?

SYMPATHETIC
Mobilised, fight or flight, angry, distressed, dysregulated

What are your emotions and how does the world feel?

Which triggers typically leave you in this state?

Which glimmers help you return to the ventral state?

DORSAL VAGAL
Immobilised, shut down, collapsed, numb, fearful, burnt out

What are your emotions and how does the world feel?

Which triggers typically leave you in this state?

Which glimmers help you return to the ventral state?

Cold-water therapy

Don't be put off by thinking this is more complicated than it is. Most of us are not inclined to plunge into a cold body of water in November just yet, but there are still manageable ways to welcome this hugely beneficial practice slowly into your daily routine.

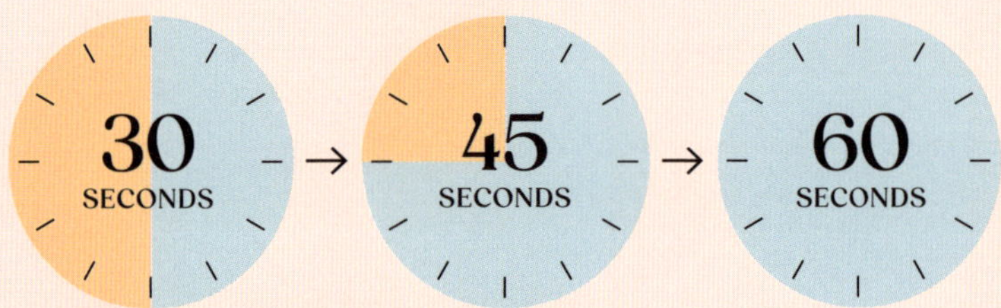

- Take a warm shower and gradually turn the tap to cold water for the last 30, 45, and then 60 seconds, building your way up. Focus on your breath and ensure you're not holding it. The more you intentionally breathe in and take long breaths out, the easier this will become. If you focus on positioning the shower head so it hits the nape of your neck, face, chest, and back, this will help activate your vagus nerve even more.
- If this feels like too much, start with your face and neck and commit to splashing them with cold water in the morning for a few seconds, building up the time each day.
- Use a cold or iced compress on your neck. Try keeping a wet flannel in a sandwich bag in the freezer for this purpose.

Strategies to take forward

Having read through this chapter, you will hopefully now feel equipped with a new understanding of your nervous system and how to work with it to move closer to safety, peace, and equilibrium. I'd like to recap on the key messages of this section.

- Remember that you no longer need to bow to neurotypical expectations: this is your chance to say when you need to decompress and unapologetically ask for what you need.
- Take time to notice the triggers telling you when you need to retreat, pause, decompress, recharge, and re-energise.
- Actively home in on uniquely identified glimmers that help soothe and relax your brain.
- Be aware somatically of what is going on in your body, and consider using grounding tools such as yoga to help you feel more present and mindful.

REFLECTIVE MOMENT

When you have the time and energy, consider these questions. They are meant to offer a gentle and safe way to explore your feelings of dysregulation and what you can do to manage them.

What trigger patterns do you begin to notice when you feel more overwhelmed and dysregulated?

What do you feel in your body when your nervous system feels compromised?

What measures are currently at your disposal to help you begin breaking these cycles?

What unique strategies have you always intuitively turned to in order to help calm and regulate your mind and body?

Which tool from this chapter may you try to deploy next time you feel dysregulated?

CHAPTER 5

Live in Sync With Your Hormones

This chapter explores the connection between ADHD and our hormones. Women are often subject to the vagaries of a monthly hormonal cycle, but how much do we know about its impact on our ADHD, and how can greater awareness help us to better manage day-to-day?

THE PROBLEM

Hormones and ADHD

I'll let you know a secret. I actually wrote this chapter last because I was overwhelmed by my ADHD and the monstrous task of tackling such a big topic. I kept wondering how I was going to fit everything I wanted to say into one chapter.

I have hours of podcasts and workshops on this topic, my own experience to reflect on, and I can observe the impact of hormones on my three neurodivergent daughters as well as my many clients. I have seen firsthand the effects hormonal fluctuations, including painful periods, PMDD, perimenopause, and menopause, have on women living undiagnosed with ADHD.

If you have experienced mental and physical health issues relating to hormonal imbalances as a neurodivergent woman, you are not alone. Research suggests that there is a significant connection between female hormones and potential neurodivergence.[26] Many of us may have gone to the doctor over and over to ask for help with heavy bleeding, mood dysregulation, anxiety, and depression, and been dismissed with some paracetamol and advice about using synthetic birth control to help 'rebalance' hormones.

PMDD & ADHD

Premenstrual Dysphoric Disorder (PMDD) is caused by an extreme drop in levels of the hormones oestrogen and progesterone after ovulation and before menstruation. We now know that there is a prevalence of PMDD in the ADHD and autistic community, with rates being nearly 50% more than for neurotypical women.[27]

BREAKING IT DOWN

The hormonal journey

From puberty through to the postmenopausal years, women spend most of their lives dealing with fluctuating hormones, and if you are living with ADHD, you might find times of hormonal change particularly challenging.

If only I knew

As with ADHD itself, everyone's journey with hormones will be different. That said, I hope that my story will resonate with many women and help to frame some common experiences. Reflect on where my story is similar to yours, where our experiences differ, and – importantly – how this makes you feel.

My hormones kicked in when I started puberty, and mood swings, anger, and extreme sensitivity began to take hold. I remember experiencing heavy periods and feeling exhausted, and thought that everyone felt their menstrual cycles so intensely that they became a different human for 7–10 days each month. The teenage years are often a heady mix of academic pressures, complicated friendships, family traumas, and lots more, so it was hard to distinguish typical angst from debilitating hormonal imbalance.

When I went to the doctor in my late teens I was given the contraceptive pill. I was told it was safe and that the worst thing that could happen would be blood clots, cramping, or mid-cycle bleeding. No doctor mentioned how the pill could make me feel more depressed, angry, and anxious than I already was, or that neurodivergence could be part of the picture. I used a wide range of birth control methods after this, but none of them agreed with me. After years of emotional upheaval, I stopped, and have since avoided synthetic hormones, knowing that they disagree with me.

When I had my first child at 25, postpartum hormones hit me like a sledgehammer, despite pregnancy having been a relatively

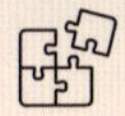

positive time. Fast-forward to 2020, in the depths of the Covid pandemic, and I was more anxious than ever before. I was overwhelmed, forgetful, and out of control. I was homeschooling four kids and launching a business while studying and coaching new clients, and I was exhausted and terrified for the future. My husband was walking on eggshells, and I wasn't sleeping properly. All the supplements I had been taking for years to keep me regulated and on a relatively even keel had stopped working.

A turning point

My doctor prescribed medication to help manage my anxiety. I picked up my prescription, yet something stopped me from taking them. I knew, that this wasn't just anxiety, there was more going on – amplified versions of something I had experienced throughout my life. A few months later, my then nine-year-old daughter was diagnosed with ADHD, and shortly after I was lucky to obtain my own diagnosis. The penny finally dropped: what was happening was a collision between ADHD and perimenopause.

There is now a lot of anecdotal evidence and new research being initiated indicating that neurodivergent women experience perimenopausal symptoms earlier than their neurotypical counterparts.[28] I wish the younger version of me had known that my brain was wired slightly differently, so I could have prepared myself for the debilitating symptoms I've experienced during times of hormonal change.

REFLECTIVE MOMENT

Pause and consider your own hormonal journey. Can you identify any times during hormonal fluctuations when your reactions and experiences have felt different or even disproportionate to other times? How, if at all, do you feel that your ADHD has played a part in this?

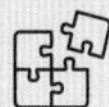

The connection between ADHD and hormones

ADELE WIMSETT, leading women's health and hormones practitioner

" A woman's brain is covered in hormone receptors for oestrogen and progesterone. If a cell has a receptor on it, it means that the cell depends on that hormone to do its job properly. When considering the executive function, cognitive function, mood regulation, sleep, and energy issues that ADHD women have, it seems absurd that hormones are not included as an integral part of managing their traits.

It is no coincidence that we see increasing numbers of women being diagnosed with ADHD at phases of their lives when hormones shift – most notably puberty, perimenopause, and menopause. Postnatally, ADHD women are also at high risk of traits flaring up. This is really important, as we know that the gender bias in research (where men have predominantly been researched and women excluded from studies on ADHD) is significant, as men do not experience these distinct hormonal life phases or fluctuations throughout the month, their hormones are largely the same every day.

Women experience a dance of hormones throughout the month if they are naturally cycling and ovulating. The first phase (follicular) is dominated by oestrogen, which sensitises neurotransmitters, and the second phase (luteal) is dominated by progesterone (if we have ovulated), which can be challenging for some as oestrogen withdrawal can exacerbate ADHD traits. However, it is worth noting that progesterone can act as a powerful mood stabiliser and have a calming impact on the nervous system, but it is often misunderstood, with many women believing they are sensitive to it. This ebb and flow also impacts the effectiveness of medication.

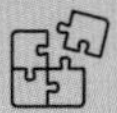

The small amount of research we currently have on ADHD and women's hormones suggests that ADHD women are at much greater risk of PMDD, postnatal depression, and of experiencing a more challenging perimenopause.[29] *Anecdotally, in my clinical experience, I also see a link with polycystic ovary syndrome (PCOS) and endometriosis, but we need more research to support this.*

I believe that the impact female hormones have on ADHD traits influences why women tend to have a delay in diagnosis. We are more likely to have our traits written off as being 'just hormonal imbalances', often feeling gaslit and alone in our experience, and some women are even misdiagnosed with anxiety or depression.

When oestrogen is high in the follicular phase, our coping strategies tend to work better. Then the luteal phase starts, and life can feel overwhelming as traits flare up, but as we enter the new cycle and oestrogen begins to rise again, we just put it down to having had a bad week. Women can spend decades in this pattern before realising that their hormones are affecting their traits. It is not until it feels like the lid has finally come off, hormonally, usually during perimenopause, that women seek support.

I believe that for women to be able to manage their ADHD traits properly, our hormones MUST be taken into consideration. Oestrogen plays a significant role in how ADHD affects a female brain from puberty to menopause, and while we do not currently have any large-scale studies on this subject, we do have surveys of women with ADHD and anecdotal experience from clinical practice indicating that oestrogen plays an important role in how ADHD brains work.

”

SCAFFOLDING TO BUILD YOU UP

Knowledge is power

If you are struggling with hormones and ADHD, know that you are not alone. There is more and more research coming to the fore as we work to understand the close connection between hormones and neurodivergence in women.

The gender health gap

Women have long been under-researched and under-prioritised in medicine. According to a report from the World Economic Forum and the McKinsey Health Institute, women spend 25% more of their lives with debilitating health than men.[30] Not only this, but medical gaslighting of women has been part of society for millennia, with 72% of women feeling like they have been medically dismissed and invalidated at some time,[31] and ADHD underdiagnosis in women definitely forms part of this picture. It's time to change the story and insist upon funding research into how conditions specifically affect women, disseminating that information to clinicians and using it to help us build up a fuller sense of our own experience.[32]

Throughout history women have had to relinquish their power to (usually male) doctors who, either from a place of ignorance or arrogance, haven't listened to or believed them. And because the research and clinical evidence hasn't existed, there has previously been little impetus to engage in further study or explore new possibilities linking women's mental, hormonal, and physical health. A woman's quality of life should never be an afterthought, and it's time we insisted that personalised and patient-centred care be made a priority.

IN HER SHOES

I thought I had PMDD for a long time and then realised that it was all ADHD-related. My periods were so bad, I would feel almost suicidal, and my hormonal changes are still an issue now, I just have more tools to help deal with them.

Allie, 41

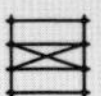

Be your own advocate

Many of us are now working hard to close the gender health gap, but until things change, the next best thing is self-empowerment and learning to advocate for yourself. This means becoming an expert on your own health, researching and homing in on your different symptoms, and not being afraid to speak up when seeing your doctor or to ask for a second opinion. Although it may sometimes seem like no one will listen, there are open-minded and passionate medical practitioners out there who are desperate to make headway in this area quickly. Please don't feel despondent – and don't stay quiet.

Keep talking

When you find a doctor or other health professional who really listens, keep an open dialogue with them. The best doctors I've met use their patients to learn and evolve. While medication and lifestyle changes help, the biggest shift comes when someone validates and understands you. Receiving recognition and compassion for a lifelong debilitating condition that has never been acknowledged before helps to remove the heavy weight we have been carrying all our lives. Knowledge and awareness are our power, and I encourage everyone to do research for themselves and print it out to present to their doctor if they think that the doctor might not be familiar with the up-to-date evidence. No matter our age or symptoms, it's important to understand the connection between ADHD, hormones, and our menstrual cycles to get the support and treatment that we need.

My dream would be an awareness poster in doctors' surgeries, detailing all the many ways a doctor could pick up on ADHD in girls so we can start supporting the next generation from a younger age.

Menopause and ADHD

DR EMMA PING, accredited menopause doctor specialising in ADHD

> *Higher oestrogen can help with mood, emotional regulation, and executive functioning, so some women with ADHD feel at their most productive and motivated during the first two weeks of their menstrual cycle, when oestrogen is higher. The menopause is diagnosed once a woman has not had a natural period for 12 months and the ovaries produce very little oestrogen or progesterone after this point. The perimenopause can last for up to 10 years prior to this, and during this time the ovaries produce oestrogen erratically and less and less leading up to menopause.*
>
> *The perimenopause is when hormones change, sometimes dramatically, and can be a turbulent time for ADHD women. The average age of menopause in the UK is 51, however, more than 1 in 100 women will reach it under the age of 40, and around 1 in 1000 below the age of 30.*[33] *A survey of 1500 women with ADHD in 2023 found that 94% reported worsening symptoms during perimenopause and menopause; a second survey in 2024 found 50% of women with ADHD experience 'life altering symptoms' in perimenopause and 83% developed new ADHD symptoms.*[34]
>
> *Many women notice that their ADHD can be more challenging during times of lower oestrogen. Women may report low mood, irritability, poorer focus, reduced memory capacity, and anxiety. Some women in perimenopause and menopause notice such a dramatic change that they fear they are developing dementia. These effects can lead to women being more vulnerable to overwhelm and burnout at this time. Others, who are taking ADHD medication, notice it is not working as effectively as before. By midlife many women with ADHD have created 'workarounds' to manage life, but during perimenopause they find these coping mechanisms are no longer effective. In reality, there are many options for addressing these changes and ADHD needs to be considered when deciding what might be right for a woman.*

Hormones and nutrition

LUCINDA MILLER, clinical lead of NatureDoc

“*Women with ADHD often face worsening symptoms during times of hormonal change. In perimenopause, the first hormone to decline is often progesterone. This can lead to anxiety, irritability, brain fog, and disturbed sleep. Declining oestrogen also affects dopamine levels, as well as the neurotransmitter GABA, which helps maintain a sense of calm.*

The right nutrition can help you manage these hormonal fluctuations and rebuild your confidence in your incredible ADHD brain. Here are my key nutritional tips:

- *Increase protein intake: Protein supports optimal brain function and can also help stabilise blood sugar levels, preventing you from feeling hangry and scattered.*

- *Reduce sugar: Consuming too much can cause fluctuations in blood sugar levels, leading to brain fog and forgetfulness.*

- *Feed your gut microbiome: Supporting gut health with a diet rich in diverse fruits, vegetables, pulses, and fermented foods like yoghurt and kefir can help you feel better balanced.*

- *Iron: Essential for making enough dopamine and deficiency can lead to brain fog. Include iron-rich foods like red meat, leafy greens, eggs, and pulses.*

- *B vitamins: Supports cognitive function and can help prevent memory loss. These come from eating meat and green veggies as well as pulses and eggs.*

- *Magnesium: Helps stabilise neurotransmitters and regulates blood sugar, which in turn can prevent brain fog and irritability. Think dark chocolate, green veggies, nuts, and seeds.*

- *Omega-3: Found in oily fish such as salmon, mackerel, and sardines, omega-3 is a brain food that supports brain cell flexibility (and thus cognitive flexibility) and executive function.*”

TOOLS TO HELP

Care for your ADHD and your menstrual cycle

These are strategies to help you curate your life and manage your ADHD in line with your menstrual cycle. This is key to understanding how your needs may vary across a month. The basic elements of a regular cycle[35] are as follows.

Menstrual phase

This is the bleed, the phase when oestrogen and progesterone are at their lowest and neurotransmitter activity is reduced. We know that this is when our ADHD traits and emotional dysregulation can be exacerbated, and the effectiveness of ADHD medication is often felt to decrease.[36] The co-occurring traits of our ADHD, such as anxiety, lack of sleep, RSD, impulsivity, brain fog, and mood regulation may also be significantly affected, causing us to feel at our worst with our ADHD symptoms and energy.[37] However, the bleed can feel like a release and a relief to many of us who have felt they have been held back by tension and stress.

Follicular phase

We're now moving out of the 'danger zone' and potentially feeling more level-headed. Our energy and focus may be improving because our oestrogen levels are rising and our progesterone remains low. This is typically when our ADHD traits don't feel as heavy and we can move through life with more ease and flow. The now increased neurotransmitter activity helps to improve mood and overall wellbeing.[38] This is a good time to see friends, book meetings, exercise, and get those trickier jobs in the diary.

Ovulatory phase

Even though we are at the peak phase of our oestrogen and may feel highly energised, this is also the top of the rollercoaster where we have all the dopamine and adrenaline but know there's going to be an extreme drop. Many neurodivergent women begin to struggle just after ovulation. This sharp fall in oestrogen coupled with rising progesterone post-ovulation can begin to exacerbate our ADHD symptoms, with some women feeling more anxious, irritable, low in energy, and experiencing low mood and lack of focus.[39]

Luteal phase

The most challenging phase for those of us with ADHD. This is because there is a steep decline in oestrogen (reducing our mood-lifting dopamine input) and a rise in progesterone. For some women, progesterone's mood-altering effects can interact negatively with stimulants and oestrogen, which means if we take daily medication the dose may need tweaking or supplementing with other medication to help move through this phase. This is especially important if PMDD has historically been a debilitating challenge.[40]

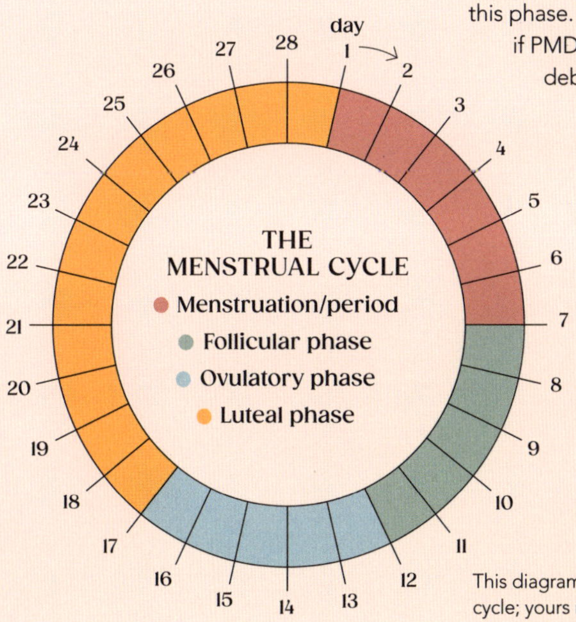

This diagram is based on an average 28-day cycle; yours might be shorter or longer.

Menstrual symptom tracker

Make a copy of this and tick off each time you experience these symptoms throughout the month.

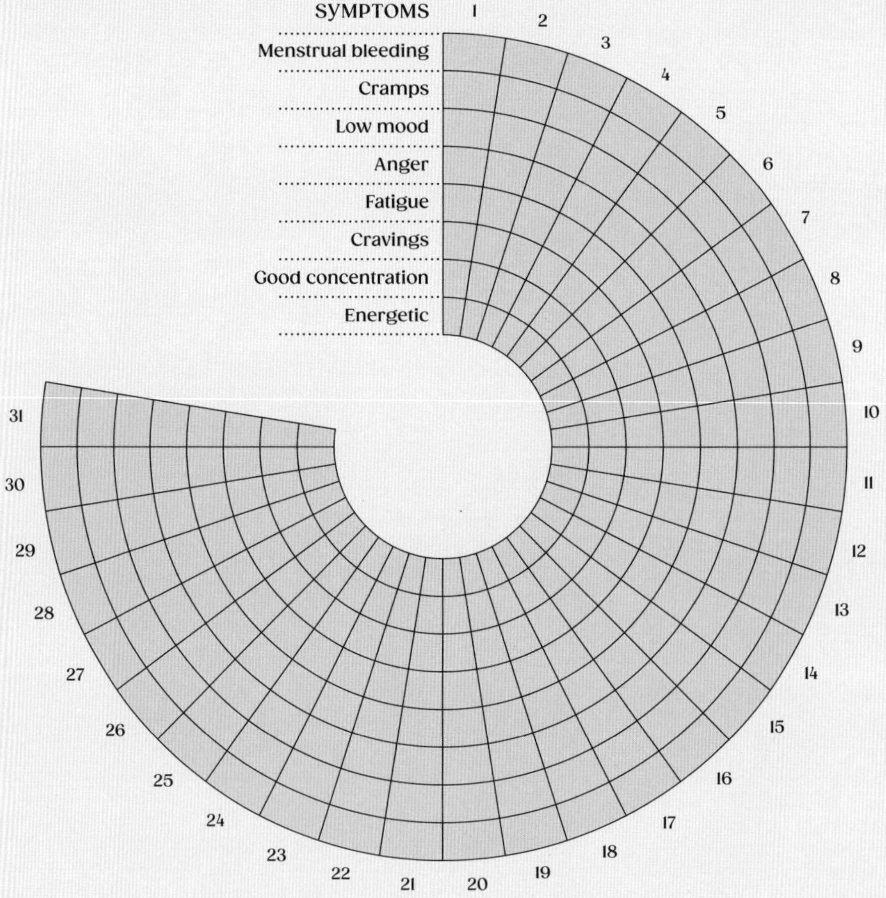

Track your cycle

By tracking your cycle, you can begin to recognise how your hormones impact your energy, mood, appetite, sleep, and focus. You can then understand how this impacts your ADHD and create strategies and structures that support you. Download an app, keep a cycle journal, make a copy of the chart opposite, or simply use your phone's notes to jot down the monthly occurrences you notice. This awareness is key, and will be a code to unlocking which triggers make your cycle harder to bear. Once you've played detective and created more of an understanding around your unique cycle – including mood, energy, cravings, sleep, sensitivities, blood loss, and pain – you can begin curating a plan that supports and enables you to thrive and not merely survive from month to month.

Plan your social life to fit your cycle

When you notice your mood and energy crashing, and that this is a monthly occurrence around the middle of your cycle, you can make decisions that will keep this time easier and calmer. Pull back from big social plans (unless they energise or uplift you), hold off from a busy working schedule, if at all possible, and begin prioritising self-care habits and gentle movement.

Ensure you have diary buffers during your more vulnerable days and weeks to give yourself space to actively replenish energy. Add some diary reminders to prepare you for the more sensitive days so they don't surprise you each month.

Recognise that your RSD (see pp.46–63) will feel more profound in the last (luteal) stage of your cycle, so offer yourself more self-understanding, self-compassion, and self-forgiveness. Educate your loved ones, too, so they know to go easy on you and recognise certain triggers around this time frame.

Look after your wellbeing

Here are my top tips for prioritising your health in line with your menstrual cycle.

- In the first week to 10 days of your cycle, when you're more energised and uplifted, consider batch-cooking any hearty meals you typically crave.
- Prioritise sleep in the vulnerable luteal week, especially as this is when we feel hotter, more restless, and more irritable (ironically, as this is when we need sleep the most). Focus on sleep hygiene as well as hydration, nutritious food, and gentle movement. Being mindful about screentime and alcohol intake can help improve sleep quality.
- Supplements have long been a lifeline for me, and I take them regularly as well as trying to eat healthily. They are beneficial for my mental health, energy, mood, and sleep. Magnesium is excellent for calming and can be taken throughout the month to help prevent extreme mood fluctuations. B vitamins are good for helping with energy, mood, cognition, and nervous system regulation. I also prioritise iron and zinc to help with brain fog and energy levels. It is important to note that supplements can interact with certain medications and you should always consult your doctor before taking any.

The more that women take note of the ebb and flow of their cycle, leaning in instead of hating or dreading it, the more life can feel like an opportunity to rest, recharge, recalibrate, and rejuvenate.

Strategies to take forward

As we've seen, hormonal fluctuations can have a huge impact on how we experience our ADHD. If this is information that you are hearing for the first time, years into adulthood, you may experience grief for all the times you have struggled in the past. This is normal. Be kind to yourself and, when you're ready, regroup and consider how you can use this knowledge to help yourself in the future.

- Try to take some time to understand your monthly cycle and to identify how it interplays with your ADHD – remember that knowledge is power.
- Show yourself kindness and compassion when you are feeling at a low ebb, and make positive decisions to protect your energy, time, and health.
- Recognise that your needs may change across your lifespan, and seek help and support when you need it.
- Guard your boundaries even more closely, upholding where you want to exert your precious energy and letting go of people or activities that deplete you.

REFLECTIVE MOMENT

When we understand the phases of our cycle, we can be more accepting and mindful of our emotions and more intentional with our actions. We can consciously choose healthier lifestyle habits or practices that intuitively feel good to us during these different phases, and move with the ebb and flow of our fluctuating and evolving cycles. When we listen to our bodies we can create a better quality of life that works for our individual needs. If you haven't tracked your cycle before, take some time now to consider the best way for you to do it. You don't have to wait for the start of a new month – you can begin tracking right now.

CHAPTER 6

Prevent Burnout

Now we'll look at how our energy stores are different from those of our neurotypical peers, often depleting faster and for varying reasons. We'll explore how to master our energy in a way that's sustainable and identify and prevent periods of burnout.

THE PROBLEM

How to identify and prevent periods of burnout

If you are living with ADHD, you're more likely to experience burnout than your neurotypical peers. But before we delve into why, let's examine what it means to 'burn out'.

Burnout is more than just having a bad day, it's a debilitating state of exhaustion: physical, mental, and emotional. It can result in the inability to cope with stimuli and a loss of skills,[41] and is more common among the neurodivergent population.[42] In fact, research suggests that adults with ADHD are three to six times more likely to experience multiple burnouts.[43] It is often brought on by a lack of awareness of our unique needs and putting other people's demands ahead of our own.

Perhaps you've never recognised your own burnout cycles, and have framed them with shame and guilt for not being able to cope with life like others around you. Right now is the moment to drop this self-blame and judgement, find self-compassion, and finally understand why you have experienced these cycles throughout life. Since my own diagnosis I have developed better tools and improved self-awareness to spot the signs of burnout before it steamrolls my life.

CHRONIC BURNOUT

Isolated episodes of burnout can be exhausting, but if they are repeated, the chronic stress that the body is under can lead to serious medical issues such as depression, cardiovascular disease, migraines, gut issues, fatigue, chronic pain, and autoimmune conditions where the body is actively fighting against its environment.[44]

BREAKING IT DOWN

Behind the burnout

Let's take a look at why burnout cycles are frequently experienced by women with ADHD.

The burnout cycle

While everyone is guilty of occasionally overworking, our ADHD brains tend to hyperfocus, which often leads to us working in a way that is exhausting and unsustainable in the long term. We are passionate and purpose-driven people, and with this comes the psychological pressure of trying to do it all, all the time.

We may also be perfectionists, with an overwhelming desire to please others, driving us to seek approval and avoid criticism at all costs. We overcompensate by always going the extra mile to meet the lofty expectations we've set ourselves. Despite this, we never feel like we achieve much and are riddled with imposter syndrome. We are never relaxed, and always feel like we should be doing something more productive.

All of this overworking and overcompensating is made even harder because of our neurodiverse executive function and working memory challenges. We can forget basics, like hydrating, eating, and fresh air, and struggle with time management so are constantly clock-watching. Task switching and interruptions can also cause a low-level hum of anxiety that is subtle but prevalent enough to make us snappy, impatient, and irritable with the people we value most. All of this can cause us to become overwhelmed and leave tasks until the very last minute. Procrastination often causes even more anxiety, and the stress from an overactive brain can affect memory and attention to detail, too. It's a self-perpetuating cycle of stress, worry, internal criticism, and shame.

IN HER SHOES

I've definitely experienced burnout. I had my own business, and I put everything into making it a success. But the stress of trying to do everything at work and at home all got too much and I started getting ill. In the end, I decided to close my business, even though I had put so much into it.

Jen, 57

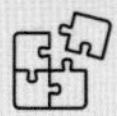

Breaking the cycle

We need to be aware of the self-perpetuating cycles that are leading us to burnout. We may enjoy our ADHD enthusiasm, wanting to do and achieve it all – but look at some of the challenges we're up against. Our expectations of what we 'should' be doing are out of alignment with what we can realistically achieve with our time, current responsibilities, and dopamine levels. Our bodies and nervous systems can't keep up with our restless, whirling minds. How could they?

We need to learn how to slow down and remember that our sensitive systems need frequent rest and recharging to function at their best. We don't question needing to recharge our phones, laptops, and cars, so why do we question ourselves for needing to rest, decompress, and have a day off? Our energy and our nervous systems have to be nurtured or we become depleted. We can resist this need and keep falling into these boom-and-bust cycles, or we can start sending ourselves some love and then tweaking our lives to work in alignment with our nervous systems.

REFLECTIVE MOMENT

Pause and read back through the challenges outlined on these two pages. What resonates with you? Can you recognise any of these experiences from your own life?

SCAFFOLDING TO BUILD YOU UP

Preserving our energy

To prevent future episodes of burnout, it's time to start thinking about our energy: why we lack it, where it comes from, and how we can preserve it.

Understand your unique energy

Our energy can be absorbed or sucked out of us in a way that is incomprehensible to a neurotypical. We surge with it on some days, hardly sitting down, but on other days we have barely enough energy to get dressed. We must learn to recognise our unique energy capacity, noticing our behaviour patterns, sleep, movement, and hormonal cycles, and be aware of what depletes and energises us. Recognising our social, sensory, physical, and emotional bandwidth and honouring our boundaries can help us more than we think. Focus on what is within your power to change, and ignore the rest. For anything you can alter, spend time considering what you can release, and what might replace it: can you visualise new ways of working, living, and being?

Energy audit

When we're depleted, we can't keep endlessly creating more energy, but we do get to choose how we utilise the energy we have and decide how to put it to the best possible use. Yes, it

Knowing your limits and capacity isn't a sign of failure or weakness, it's a recognition of self-respect and self-preservation.

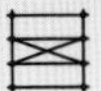

may not be fair that we can't throw our energy around regardless of the repercussions the next day, but this allows us to be intentional with every decision we make, curating a healthier and more authentic way of being for ourselves and our families.

When we know our energy is dipping, learning to ask for what we need or instilling boundaries without fear of catastrophised repercussions is crucial. We need to offer this to ourselves without fear or judgement. We should also be proactive about staging personal audits and interventions, because as burnout hits, it can become harder to recognise what is happening.

Find your energy equilibrium

It is empowering to know that you can be the architect of your energy field, and of your life. The more you step into your power to make choices that are right for you, but which may not suit those around you, the more you'll notice your energy equilibrium. You won't experience the intense surges and dips as much, and you'll have more respect and kindness for yourself when you do need to rest. As ADHDers, we are used to the boom-bust cycle, where one day's high intensity can lead to sheer exhaustion and inability to act the next. What we're aiming for is something much more balanced – not a total eradication of highs and lows, as that would be impossible (and boring!), but by reducing the pendulum swing to a more manageable level, where there may be better and worse days, you'll be able to cope and move forward steadily.

REFLECTIVE MOMENT

Pause and consider your emotional, social, spiritual, and physical energy levels: where, when, and with whom are these being used up the most? Think of yourself as a bucket with holes, and your energy as water draining away – where are these holes, what form do they take, and how can you begin mending each one?

Ask for help

Taking care of ourselves doesn't always come easily. Despite finding it difficult to prioritise tasks due to my ADHD executive functioning challenges, I'm learning how to ask for help and delegate jobs that feel depleting to create more space to do things I enjoy, which don't completely drain me, and I know I am good at.

Asking for help is a game-changer (but also difficult if you've been brought up not feeling safe or if you always had to be the capable one), and when you do this, try to be as specific as you can. Consider what assistance you could ask for. It doesn't need to be paid help, and you shouldn't feel guilty about seeking it; we may be used to being someone else's 'super-helper', but we're deserving of help, too.

Tackle 'brain-heavy' tasks

On the whole, to get brain-heavy tasks done, I have to do them my way, riding the waves of adrenaline and dopamine. Sometimes I use my 'brain-heavy' strategy, but I use it intentionally and I know how to take extra care of myself when it is happening. To tackle 'brain-heavy' tasks in this way, ask yourself the following questions.

- Is this something that needs to be done straight away? Or can it wait and be filed for a later date?
- Am I medicated (maybe caffeinated) and nutritionally nourished, and have I slept enough to tackle this task?
- Am I interested or motivated to do this right now?
- Do I have the energy stores to do this right now?
- Can I redirect myself to something that needs my attention more (this may be allowing myself time to rest)?

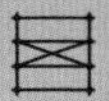

Give some thought to your answers (and be honest). If the task is something that needs to be done and you're enthusiastic and feel you have the energy to do it, then just go for it. In this case, make sure that you have allowed time afterwards to recuperate. If the task doesn't need to be completed immediately, ask yourself whether you can redirect your energy to something else, and if you're already feeling depleted, prioritise rest and relaxation. It may not work every time, but the more that you can practise mindfully engaging with tasks, the easier this process will become.

Build in recuperation time

Something that has helped me over the past few years is understanding my patterns and acknowledging that if I have powered through using my reserves to get over the line, I need to recognise the toll it takes on me afterwards and prepare for this. So instead of scheduling in another similar day straight after, I accept that if I have a crazy day or two (and depending on where I am in my menstrual cycle), as a non-negotiable I book in enough space and decompression time to recover. Being intentional with recovery time is vital for neurodivergent people. This strategy helps us recentre and ground ourselves instead of self-sabotaging all our ambitions and plans with a constant cycle of burnout.

We have to acknowledge that our energy is finite. This is true for everyone, but especially so for those of us with ADHD. We can't give what we don't have: that leads to burnout.

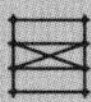

The importance of gut health for our brain and energy levels

DR GEMMA NEWMAN, doctor, speaker, and the author of *Get Well, Stay Well* and *The Plant Power Doctor*

“Gut health is one of the newest trends in wellness, and you will probably have noticed an explosion of products on the market touted as being good for your gut, or that contain ‘gut friendly’ bacteria. The word ‘microbiome’ is also becoming more widely recognised. But what is the significance of having a healthy gut microbiome, and what on earth does this have to do with maintaining a healthy brain?

The gut microbiome is a vast array of bacteria, viruses, and parasites that create an ecosystem within us. It has distinct functions that support our health in many ways. For optimal health, researchers agree that we should have many varieties of beneficial bacteria in our large intestine. We keep them alive as their host, and in return they work for us, breaking down fibres and plant nutrients that our bodies can use for gut lining, properly absorbing nutrients, and preventing infections and autoimmune over-reactivity. They even help us with mood and brain functioning.

Fibre from foods like fruits, vegetables, peas, beans, tofu, lentils, and wholegrains are not only healthy for us, but they are also how we feed our healthy gut bugs. When these foods are broken down in our intestine by bacteria, substances called Short Chain Fatty Acids (SCFAs) are produced. These are truly amazing molecules, because they help the gut lining remain strong, thus reducing the risk of inflammatory bowel disorders or unwanted exposure to toxins from the environment that pass through our guts. SCFAs have powerful calming effects on our immune function, too. They are potentially helpful in reducing the risk of a number of immune mediated conditions, from eczema and psoriasis to MS and lupus. They also have anti-cancer effects, and reduce our chances of developing obesity and type 2 diabetes.

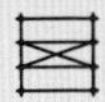

Eating fibre-rich foods acts as the perfect prebiotic (food for your microbes). Meanwhile, eating fermented foods can provide probiotics (beneficial microbes). Examples of foods that already contain beneficial bugs include yogurt, kimchi, miso, and sauerkraut.

Just as SCFAs help to protect the intestinal barrier, they can also protect the blood–brain barrier. This is an important way to protect the brain itself from unwanted toxic metabolites and inflammation. SCFAs have been detected in the fluid that surrounds the brain, and they also seem to have a role in the healthy development of microglial cells. Microglial cells are the most important immune cells of the central nervous system and are the first to respond when something goes wrong in the brain. Alterations in both dopamine levels and microglial activation have been shown to be linked to ADHD.

SCFAs can provide energy for the brain, and they have been shown to affect the function of neurons, including helping us to consolidate long-term memories. SCFAs also have a role in controlling neurons, which can in turn impact our appetite control and day–night (circadian) rhythm. This is all very relevant when it comes to ADHD, as many with ADHD report difficulties with memory, sleeping, and appetite regulation.

It is possible that enjoying foods that allow SCFAs to flourish in our guts is an important way for the gut–brain connection to help improve brain function. A recent study showed that people with ADHD tend to have lower levels of SCFAs in their bloodstream than non-ADHD controls, and that the levels of SCFAs were also impaired by taking antibiotics and being on stimulant medication. It is not possible to draw solid conclusions from this research, and I do not recommend coming off stimulant medication if you feel it is working well for you, or avoiding antibiotics if you need them, but this research helps us to begin making links between things we can do to improve our general and brain health.[45] ”

TOOLS TO HELP

Nurture your energy stores

Here are some practical tools that will help you to avoid burnout and manage your valuable – and finite – energy stores.

Restore your energy stores

A simple way to build your energy stores is to take note of when your body and mind feel rested: what have you been doing? Who have you been with? Track and record the days in this way. Take an inventory for a few weeks and see how you feel at the end of each day. Tally up the activities, the people, the rest, the movement, the food, the fun, and see what you can do more of. Create a personalised ADHD formula that works fluidly for you. This is the beginning of curating a life that works on your terms.

Everyone charges up their energy batteries differently. The result is what matters: if it works for you, then it is right for you. Some ways I like to build up my energy stores with the time I have at my disposal include the following.

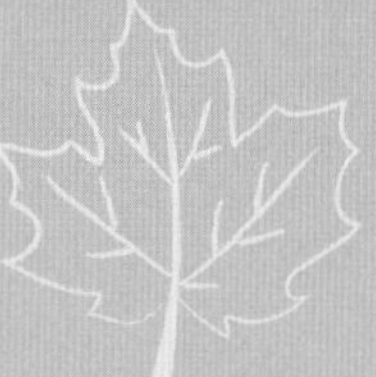

Walking in nature with my dog, listening to nothing but the outdoors, a good podcast, or music without self-judgement.

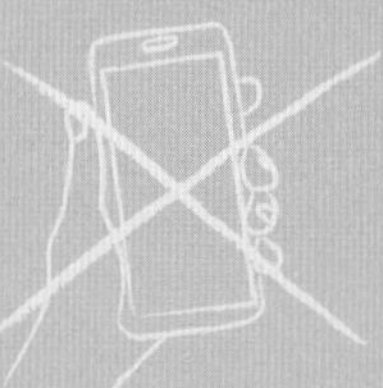

Phone-free time: I put my phone away and my energy is restored; no pings, notifications, or sense of urgency to check emails or social media updates.

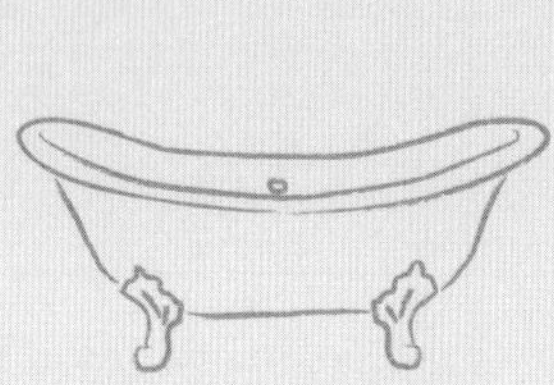

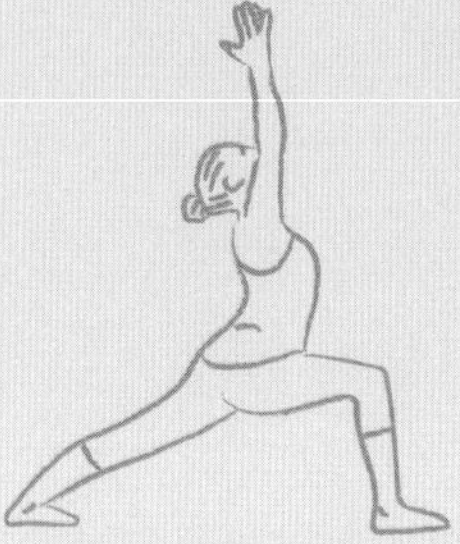

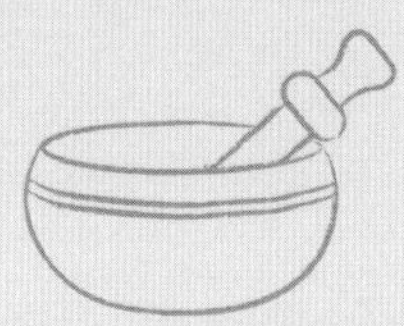

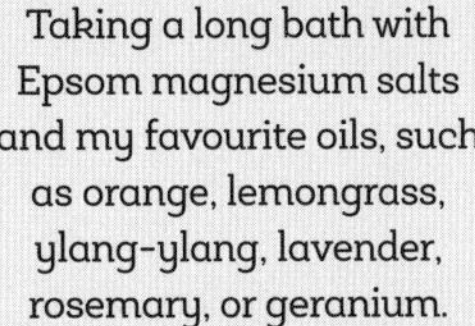

Taking a long bath with Epsom magnesium salts and my favourite oils, such as orange, lemongrass, ylang-ylang, lavender, rosemary, or geranium.

Doing yoga or gentle stretching, anything slow and restorative with long poses, lots of breathwork, and space to relax.

Listening to Binaural beat music or going to gong or sound baths calms my nervous system, allows my mind to rest, and helps me feel more energised.

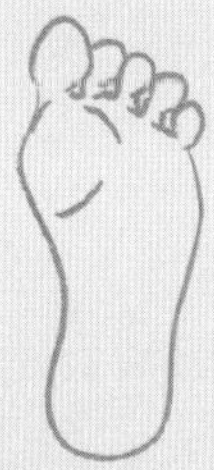

Having a meaningful chat or walk with a friend who just 'gets me', and vice versa.

Reflexology – this is my favourite way to experience a feeling of instant relaxation.

Recognise your burnout signs

The first step to managing burnout is learning about the warning signs your body displays. Spotting these early will help you to put your prevention plan in place in good time. Create a checklist with these items on and run through it each day.[46]

EMOTIONAL SIGNS OF BURNOUT	M	T	W	T	F	S	S
feeling tired or drained most of the time							
becoming overwhelmed							
feeling like dropping it all and running away							
feeling detached and/or lonely							
disconnecting from friends and family							
thinking constant negative thoughts							
feeling on edge or anxious							

PHYSICAL SIGNS OF BURNOUT	M	T	W	T	F	S	S
headaches and migraines							
sleep issues or insomnia							
ongoing back/neck/ shoulder pain							
chronic gut issues							
lowered immunity or recurrent illness							
jaw ache and clenching							

Create a burnout-prevention plan

Creating a plan that you can print out and easily refer to can be useful. You can build on this over time as you identify more of the signs that show you're moving into a burnout phase. It's a good idea to share your plan with loved ones, so they can help you to spot the early signs as well. Your plan could include the following.

1. ***Warning signs:*** you can pull these in from the exercise on the opposite page, and add any extras you spot too; for example, extreme phone use and social media scrolling, eating less, losing interest in exercise, and not wanting to talk to friends and family. Make a note of the time of the month when these happen and any other details about the experience, such as what you have been doing around the time these signs appear.

2. ***Triggers:*** after mapping when you experience burnout signs, look for what connects the episodes. This will help you to establish the things that you know cause you to feel burnt out; for example, a clash of social and work commitments.

3. ***Patterns:*** are there any patterns across the month or months? This may help you to identify any hormonal underpinnings.

SET UP AN EMERGENCY BURNOUT BOX

You could consider creating an 'emergency box' that you can easily access if you feel yourself struggling. This box could include things that can provide shortcuts and help you reduce the executive functioning needed to access activities that you find restorative, with items such as Epsom salts, essential oils, herbal teas, a weighted blanket, and some TV programme ideas that calm your brain and nervous system.

Harnessing future wisdom

Using future wisdom helps us see what's ahead, when typically we go full-steam in the moment, committing to arrangements and saying yes far too often. Future-proofing yourself is integral to preventing burnout and overwhelm cycles because it allows you to be one step ahead of your impulsive, excited, and curious self. Here are a few ideas for how to use future wisdom.

Every week, check your diary and commitments. Ensure you have buffers in place and space in between so timing doesn't make you anxious and you have time to yourself to unwind.

Say no. You will still be liked, and potentially respected even more, if you say no more than yes.

Remember: cancelling plans is not a crime.

Schedule in time to decompress, literally write 'decompression' as well as putting energising time-blocks in your diary so you aren't running on empty.

Check your sensory outputs: what is it that overloads your system? Is it noises, smells, light, or voices?

Strategies to take forward

- Try to spot your subtle burnout signs early and assemble some tried-and-tested tools so that when you do feel your energy levels dipping, you can take speedy action.
- Aim to have firm boundaries around people, situations, and environments that deplete your energy: you don't have to always say yes and people-please anymore.
- Delegate tasks you find difficult instead of persevering with them: there's no shame in asking for help where you struggle, allowing you to focus on the areas where you really shine.
- Don't forget the importance of lifestyle improvements and tweaks such as prioritising sleep, spending time outdoors in daylight, daily movement, and healthy eating choices, and recognise the mind–gut connection when it comes to maintaining energy levels.

REFLECTIVE MOMENT

We can also lean into our hormonal cycles to avoid burnout. You will recall from chapter 5 that we gain an energy boost in the first half of our menstrual cycle (the follicular phase, when oestrogen rises in the first 10–14 days). This is the time to do 'big things'.

As we move to the second half of our cycle (the luteal phase, when oestrogen drops and progesterone begins to increase), and on towards menstruation (when both oestrogen and progesterone drop), energy ebbs again and we should pull back from demanding commitments, keep watch of our boundaries and allow ourselves to retreat with self-compassion.

Recognising that we have these ebbs and flows allows us to slow down and acknowledge that we don't need to be 'on' all the time. Reflect on how you can factor hormonal changes into your monthly schedule and burnout prevention plan.

CHAPTER 7

Build a Life That Works for You

You might have spent years masking your ADHD, and living in a way that feels authentic may have felt beyond your reach. Here, we'll explore how you can gently leave those days behind and get curious about curating a life that works for you, where your ADHD can become a strength rather than a mystery force that's holding you back.

THE PROBLEM

Harnessing your ADHD

If you've been living with ADHD, especially if it's gone undiagnosed, you'll likely be in basic survival mode. You may be doing what you need to do to get by and questioning yourself at every turn – but there is a better way.

Living in a way that doesn't suit us can feel suffocating and uninspiring. Many of us live with a constant self-critical narrative, thinking everything is entirely within our control and yet never understanding why we behave as we do. It takes time to shed lifelong beliefs that leave us feeling less than, but if you can commit to a small act each day to break them down, you'll soon look back at the old version of yourself and see progress.

It's time to begin a new chapter by creating a compassionate, ADHD-informed blueprint for a new version of yourself, one that embraces your integral values, deep desires, and conscious choices. Questions to ask yourself as we begin this chapter are:

- In the different areas of your life, such as friendships, career, and energy, what are you not willing to accept anymore?
- What boundaries are you ready to unapologetically put in place?
- What are you ready to let go of that has blocked you from feeling energised, grounded, centred, and balanced?

Together, we are going to embrace a shedding process to help you become the most truthful version of you who lives life imperfectly but with far more authenticity.

BREAKING IT DOWN

Reconsidering how you live

Many of us have been conditioned to think that there's a 'right' or 'wrong' way to live or linear path we must follow. But for those of us who are neurodivergent in a mostly neurotypical world, these expectations often don't fit us well.

A different way of being

I genuinely don't recognise the person I've become over the last five years. The old me never worked from a place of self-compassion, my default was always self-blame. I still have many moments of imposter syndrome and honestly wonder how I'm now here, writing a book, but I've dedicated a great deal of time to healing and grounding to get to this point. My journey hasn't been linear, and I haven't experienced one big life-changing moment. I've had many times where I've wanted to throw in the towel and self-sabotage has come knocking. But, through ongoing work on myself, I've discovered my many strengths, passions, hopes, resilience, and pride. This hasn't come from external validation, but from finally understanding myself and my wiring, plus all the conflicting parts that make me, and accepting them without judgement or shame.

I wish I'd known this back in my early 20s when, after several years of working in consumer PR, I felt more and more like an outsider. I hated working weekends with little downtime, and I didn't enjoy late-night drinking with colleagues; I was drained after working in a busy, noisy, and bright office. Even then I knew that what I really needed was a hot bath and a TV dinner. I had sensory differences and craved fresh air, natural light, walks, and water for my wellbeing before I knew what any of this meant.

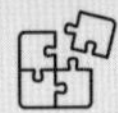

You haven't understood yourself because you have a neurobiological difference that you knew nothing about. When you don't have a roadmap, it's difficult to know where to go.

When I got married at the very young age of 23 and had a baby at 25, I was treated as though I'd decided to join a cult or live on an island in the South Pacific. No one got that I wanted a simpler life (not quite what happened after four kids) with fewer expectations put on me from external situations. I wanted to cultivate my own autonomy and pace of life. I liked being busy, but I hated answering to other people when my nervous system was crying out for the freedom to live on my terms.

The right conditions to thrive

When we buy a houseplant, there are always instructions on where to position it. We take notice, and pop it in a space where it will flourish. Why, as humans, do we not afford ourselves the same treatment? Why are we expected to all thrive in the same situations, and when we don't we are blamed? But we can change the story; no one tells us this, but we can. We get to look at the areas of our life that are no longer working – or perhaps never worked – and find more soul-aligned techniques. This could mean a diverse work environment, new friendships, exciting hobbies, an interesting holiday – this is our time to position ourselves wherever feels good throughout the seasons.

SCAFFOLDING TO BUILD YOU UP

Tuning in to your needs

It's time to look forward and consider how you can start really listening to your needs and begin advocating for yourself, creating better awareness of what helps you thrive and live your life more authentically.

Live intentionally

When we accept who we are and let go of expectations, we can start tuning in to what we really need. This could mean leaving an office-based corporate job and working outside in nature or from home, or recognising why the gym has always felt so arduous but outdoor swimming feels like a treat.

A great way of tuning in to our needs is by using our physical bodies to feel what works for us. Gentle and short breathwork practices once an hour can make a profound difference (see pp.60–61), as can a short walk without technology once a day. Connecting with our bodies helps us to tune in to our inner knowledge and wisdom, and that is what we need to be listening to.

Many of us haven't been taught how to listen to our bodies, and any innate awareness has been wiped out by our outdated education, stifling upbringing, and a way of life that never suited our wiring. This is a practice that takes time and patience, and a deep commitment to overriding frustration at not being able to immediately connect to this part of us. You may hear this understanding of bodily functions referred to as 'interoception'; Dr Stephen Porges, the creator of polyvagal theory (see p.72) calls interoception a 'sixth sense', as it's the means by which the body communicates its sensory needs without us being consciously aware. Our interoceptive sense is often responding to threats in our environment that we also haven't consciously recognised (something Dr Porges refers to as 'neuroception').[47]

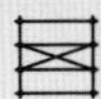

Leaning into self-trust

We all have dreams and aspirations, but when we are living with ADHD, most of the time we're too afraid to voice them aloud. A lifetime of being ridiculed, not listened to, or fearing how we communicate means we look to others for approval and validation. Neurodivergent brains are renowned for homing in on out-of-the-box perspectives – we're trailblazers, outliers, and trendspotters – and when this is celebrated and encouraged, we can further embrace this expansive thinking. However, if this has not been nurtured, or we've been taught to shrink and suppress this part of ourselves due to a need to feel safe or accepted, leaning into self-trust as opposed to the default mode of self-doubt is a terrifying suggestion.

When we haven't trusted our abilities for most of our adult lives, or have been unsure how we've achieved what we have because our methods look very different, messy, or perhaps highly unique, we instantly doubt that we have what it takes to get to where we want to be. We've already discussed imposter syndrome (see p.37), and it can take lots of self-awareness, inner work, and therapy to leave it behind and finally believe in ourselves and what we have to offer. When we can trust that we have what it takes, we begin to see a life brimming with potential and possibilities. As my confidence has grown over the past five years, from the inception of my business with its female ADHD focus, I've had to consistently and terrifyingly lean into self-trust. I knew that if I needed this information, there would be many other women in a similar situation.

IN HER SHOES

What helps? Staying out of my head. Trying to avoid situations that will upset or trigger me. Some exercise (I hate it but know I need to do some at least). Me time. Avoiding the news and any books or TV shows that will upset me. Being in the garden.

Alison 67

Flexing the self-trust muscle is a mindset gamble that mostly pays off because, even if a particular idea didn't work out, what we've learnt from going through the stages of the experience will always be worthwhile, even if it didn't quite work out the way we wanted. Over time, with our back catalogue of fear-inducing experiences, we are able to make more aligned, self-led decisions and no longer be paralysed by self-doubt. This is how we cultivate a growth mindset, which is a particularly helpful asset for those of us with ADHD.

A few questions to ask yourself when you're feeling uncertain include the following:

- What if it *did* work out?
- What's the worst that would happen if it failed or did not go according to plan?
- What signs in your body can you recognise when it's either a 'hell yeah' or a 'yuck, no'? Note these down with brief examples: such as spotting a fabulous dress, saying yes to an adventure, settling on a holiday destination, or discovering a recipe that sings to you. Notice the feelings in your body – what are you feeling when you do something fun or something against your values or interests?
- Write out affirmations such as: 'I choose to trust and believe that I have the answers within me', 'I am choosing to listen and trust my inner guidance and wisdom', and 'Even though things may not go to plan, I am always learning and growing'.

Simply listening to your body, learning and understanding its unique language, is the foundation for working with it rather than against it.

Becoming self-aware

LIDIA ZYLOWSKA M.D., ADHD and mindfulness expert and author

"Learning what ADHD is and how it can show up in one's life is very important when you first get diagnosed, so I always encourage patients to choose a book, podcast, online resource, or ADHD community that can help them understand common patterns – often those beyond typical diagnostic criteria – that appear for women. Hearing other people's stories alongside expert ADHD knowledge can help those who are newly diagnosed to recognise more fully (and put into words) their own experiences related to ADHD. This psychoeducation increases self-awareness.

The 'on-the-spot' or 'in-the-moment' awareness that mindfulness training teaches is key to a deeper understanding of yourself and your ADHD. So many ADHD behaviours or the coping strategies that evolved around them (notably, not always helpful coping strategies) happen automatically, so bringing in-the-moment curiosity and nonjudgement is vital. For example, noticing, 'I tend to feel anxious and my muscles tense up when I want to say no to a project... but I end up agreeing anyway', or 'I see how I avoid starting on any paperwork and feel tired just thinking about it'. This kind of nonjudgemental awareness often opens up opportunities to problem-solve; for example, breathing through the anxiety of saying 'no' and practising 'the gracious no', such as 'thank you for the interesting opportunity but I have too many commitments right now. Perhaps in the future'.

Many women with ADHD cope with the condition by becoming perfectionists, so it is important to have self-compassion around this. You can practise 'tuning in' to yourself to see what fears or anxieties come up when you think about perfectionism ('I am not enough' or 'I can't trust how I will show up') that can lead you to overpreparing or to self-criticism. Embracing these layers with self-compassion can help you balance striving for improvement with a more accepting relationship with yourself."

TOOLS TO HELP

Access your feelings

We will now explore some tools that will help you to tune in to your emotions and start to understand your needs on a deeper level, so you can clarify who you ultimately want to be – and discover how to get there.

Ikigai

The Japanese philosophy of ikigai promotes a way of being that's centred on living with purpose and feeling fulfilled; it offers us a reason to be here and helps us to recognise that our contribution is valuable and unique. When people tell us to find our passion and purpose, it can feel ambiguous and elusive – especially with late-diagnosed ADHD, where we might have many passions but we don't feel confident enough to lean into them. We may not even really know what our purpose is, or that we're deserving of a life that feels more enjoyable and easier. You can use this concept as an invitation to ponder on what you've been ignoring or perhaps refusing to consider.

Ikigai is based on:

- Doing what we love
- Doing what we are good at
- Doing what the world needs
- Doing what we can be paid for

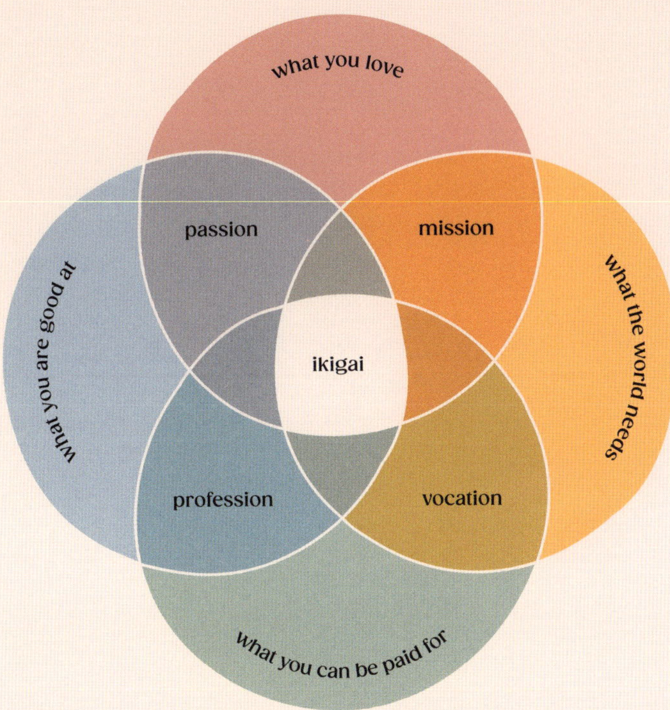

Ikigai suggests that we are able to harmonise these four components in our unique way, and at the intersection of them will find fulfilment and a more enjoyable and effortless life; one that works in synergy with our authenticity, values, strengths, talents, and interests. The ikigai framework is simple and works with our divergent thinking: we learn to identify and hone our strengths, then work on weaving them into our passions (which can change over time), leading us to our purpose.

As a starting point, you can use this diagram to help find your own ikigai. See this as a value-driven roadmap to help you identify what truly matters to you and what energises you on a soul level, while keeping it practical – enabling you to live a life more on your terms and recognising how this can be financially sustainable.

Delve deeper into your emotions

Many of us who see ourselves as neurodivergent might also identify with alexithymia, which means having difficulties with experiencing, identifying, and expressing emotions. Some estimates suggest that 41.5% of people with ADHD may also have this as a co-occurring condition.[48] If this feels like a trait you relate to, using a feelings wheel or chart can benefit both you and your relationships. It will gently guide you through your emotional state and help you identify your feelings, encouraging you to pause and reflect as you go.

Being aware of the nuances of your emotions will help you to ask for what you need, and allow you to prepare for those challenging moments where you may feel like your boundaries have been crossed. A feelings wheel, such as the one shown opposite, encourages you to delve into your emotions, their triggers, and how they feel in your body. Give yourself some time to identify those deeper emotions, and think of when you experienced them and why.

It's common for neurodivergent women to feel misunderstood and potentially gaslighted. Someone may dismiss or invalidate an RSD experience that feels very raw and real, and we may have repressed this emotion; this means we are easily triggered next time a similar situation happens, displaying what is perceived as an extreme reaction to a seemingly throwaway remark. Instead of repressing these emotions and blaming yourself for being 'too sensitive' yet again, offer yourself this space to gently recognise what happened and examine why you felt anxious, criticised, overwhelmed, or distressed that particular time.

Feelings wheel

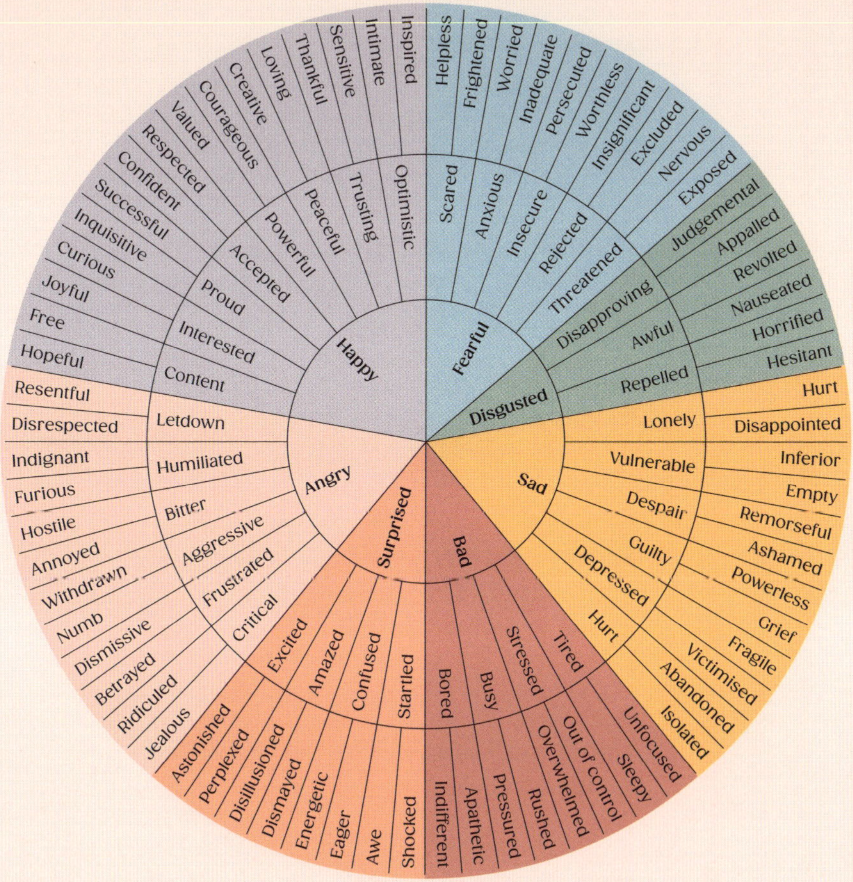

Fearful
Scared, Anxious, Insecure, Rejected, Threatened
Helpless, Frightened, Worried, Inadequate, Persecuted, Worthless, Insignificant, Excluded, Nervous, Exposed

Disgusted
Disapproving, Awful, Repelled
Judgemental, Appalled, Revolted, Nauseated, Horrified, Hesitant

Sad
Lonely, Vulnerable, Despair, Guilty, Depressed, Hurt
Hurt, Disappointed, Inferior, Empty, Remorseful, Ashamed, Powerless, Grief, Fragile, Victimised, Abandoned, Isolated

Bad
Tired, Stressed, Busy, Bored
Unfocused, Sleepy, Out of control, Overwhelmed, Rushed, Pressured, Apathetic, Indifferent

Surprised
Startled, Confused, Amazed, Excited
Shocked, Awe, Eager, Energetic, Dismayed, Disillusioned, Perplexed, Astonished

Angry
Critical, Frustrated, Aggressive, Bitter, Humiliated, Letdown
Jealous, Ridiculed, Betrayed, Dismissive, Numb, Withdrawn, Annoyed, Hostile, Furious, Indignant, Disrespected, Resentful

Happy
Content, Interested, Proud, Accepted, Powerful, Peaceful, Trusting, Optimistic
Hopeful, Free, Joyful, Curious, Inquisitive, Successful, Confident, Respected, Valued, Courageous, Creative, Loving, Thankful, Sensitive, Intimate, Inspired

Undertake a self-audit

This is a simple practice to help you identify what's going on when you are feeling overwhelmed and put more effective boundaries in place moving forward.

1 ***Identify your boundaries***

Take some time to reflect on your boundaries and what they mean to you. Note down your five non-negotiables, why they are important to you, and how you feel when they are compromised.

2 ***Identify when the expectations of others force you to compromise your boundaries***

Consider when you've compromised your boundaries, haven't clearly expressed them to others, or have allowed someone to bulldoze over them. Get specific with examples and details. It doesn't have to be one big dramatic event – a series of small, ongoing events can contribute to us feeling overwhelmed, disregarded, or burnt out.

3 ***Identify when your own expectations force you to compromise your boundaries***

It's time to also consider the expectations you put on yourself. We know there is a tendency towards perfectionism and people-pleasing in the neurodivergent community. Ask yourself if you'd put these same expectations on others, and if not, get curious about where your own conditioning has come from. When we begin breaking down old beliefs and mindsets, we can usually trace it to a childhood issue that was repressed or normalised.

Letting go of the unrealistic expectations we place on ourselves helps us to become more compassionate to those around us. It's okay to not finish all the tasks on our to-do lists, to not always have a clean home, eternally happy children, a healthy diet, organised files, and consistent friendship meetups!

Strategies to take forward

It can feel daunting to look at your life and realise that you need to make many changes in order to reach a place where your ADHD self can truly thrive. The key is to start small: each little adjustment that brings you more into alignment with yourself will help you build to a point where you feel safe, content, and able to live authentically.

- Be kind to yourself: remember that decisions you made in the past were without the knowledge you have today.
- Consider all the areas of your life in which you can make readjustments, including what you eat, where you go, and the time you offer yourself to relax. You don't have to deal with everything all at once, but looking holistically at the small details of your lifestyle can be just as important as making big changes around your job, friendships, boundaries, and relationships.
- Remind yourself that the goal is to gently curate a life that works for you, and the people who care about you will want this for you too. Trust your instincts and believe in your own power to bring about the change you need.

REFLECTIVE MOMENT

We don't get into trouble for having a good life. The joy police aren't going to take away the stuff we enjoy because we are doing too much of it. Part of curating a life that works for you means building the things that you enjoy into your day. Take a moment to think of one fun or creative activity you can do tomorrow (or even right now), something you don't normally do or haven't done in a while that will help you feel life is working with rather than against you.

CHAPTER 8

Boost Your Creativity

In this chapter we'll focus on creativity: why it's important, why it can be missing, how we can get it back, and how it can be sustained. If you're feeling creatively blocked, we're going to unpick what has been holding you back and look ahead to a more expansive future.

THE PROBLEM

Purpose anxiety and creativity

Let's first take a look at what could be preventing us from accessing our creativity, and then explore how we can harness and channel it effectively.

We've talked a lot about some of the paradoxical challenges of ADHD. In order to make the most of our fast-paced neurodivergent brains, we need to understand what can block our creativity, and how we can harness it moving forward.

Elizabeth Gilbert, journalist, speaker, and author of one of my favourite books, *Big Magic*, suggests that the pressure Western society has placed on us to believe that we're all here to share our unique purpose is just too much. It has caused us to suffer from a concept she calls 'purpose anxiety', and this is actually blocking our path to creativity.

Purpose anxiety, coupled with a heady mix of imposter syndrome, self-doubt, overwhelm, people-pleasing and perfectionist tendencies, and cognitive processing differences that many of us with ADHD experience, can block creativity before we even work up the curiosity to get started. And when you add ADHD 'all or nothing' thinking into the mix, our brains can tell us to give up before we even try, despite us probably having at least three ideas for a new creative project per week.

We need to learn ways to live in the moment and unlock our creativity, but how can we do that intentionally?

When we lean into our unique creative flow, this also helps us to think more expansively across all areas of our life.

BREAKING IT DOWN

The power of creativity

Creativity can be beneficial to our mental wellbeing and helps enormously when navigating the challenges of ADHD. It also allows us to step into a mindful and flow-like state, taking us out of our busy, restless, and must-be-productive way of being.

Relinquishing anxiety

Remember our powerful creative firelighter, the task positive network from chapter 2? Well, it is activated when we use our imagination and allow creative ideas to flow. When we power up this integral neural pathway, we keep the more negative part of our brain – the ruminating and doom-mongering default mode network (a.k.a. the demon! See p.33), from becoming too prominent a player in our daily choices. It is in this way that creativity can become a balm for some of the more challenging symptoms of ADHD. We can either choose to ruminate, worry, and catastrophise, or we can say, 'no, I'm choosing to engage my brain's wiring to create positive thoughts, energy, and action'; the easiest and fastest way to do this is by intentionally 'plugging in' the TPN and finding something creative and mindful to do.

IN HER SHOES

Thinking creatively and outside the box is a huge ADHD strength. Often, I can see the bigger picture in situations and what different possible outcomes could be. Quite often people haven't thought of some of the solutions that immediately come to mind.

Tanya, 49

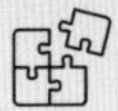

Inner clarity

Creativity can also bring a sense of inner clarity and awareness, both of which will help you feel more centred and in control (and so in a better place to manage the challenges of ADHD).

In my own life, this felt particularly apparent when I left my work in PR to launch a business selling succulents. When the kids were in bed, I would go into the back room, roll my sleeves up, and listen to music, podcasts, and audiobooks while I worked. This is what eventually piqued my interest in self-development, spirituality, coaching, and emotional wellbeing. I've never felt so aligned as when I was on this creative sabbatical. This period of my life sowed the seeds for my career as it is now; I was unknowingly creating new pathways for how I wanted to live.

Engaging in a creative pursuit that inspired me set my life off in a completely different direction, one that I wouldn't have figured out by just sitting down with pen and paper and a desire to make a plan. Our ADHD brains need to 'free flow' in the way that only creativity allows.

Accessing a flow state

Harnessing our ADHD creativity is like finally using an extra limb that used to trip us up. Of course, we can't generalise and say every person with ADHD or who relates to being neurodivergent is also a creative genius, but I like to believe that creativity lies dormant in us all. There is no one-size-fits-all way of being creative. Learning to find calm and mindful moments while we're in a creative flow state is something we can all explore, and the more we do it, the more we will realise what a wonderful tonic it is to take a break from our endless tech and social media usage. Children are our mirrors, and I see such a change in behaviour and attitude after my daughter has done some baking or artwork, away from her phone or tablet. When we put some music on, pull out the Lego, and get lost in this flow state, it's like a warm bath for our brains and nervous systems.

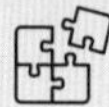

Why we're inherently creative

JUDE SCHWEPPE, performance coach, writer, actor, and co-founder of the Actors' Space in Brighton, UK

"When I look back over the meandering course of my life as a woman who spent 45 chaotic years wondering why she couldn't seem to get herself together – despite having every tool in the kit – the one thing that has been a constant source of comfort, inspiration, community, and joy is my creative practice.

I began dance classes when I was four; I sang my way through the loneliness of being an only child until my sister arrived when I was seven; I fell wildly and passionately in love with acting at the age of 12, and went on to train as an actor when I left university. I learned to DJ in my 20s, and spent several years moonlighting as a music journalist while attempting to squeeze myself into a 9–5-shaped job in advertising. And, more recently, I have returned to painting, making things, and writing for pleasure and therapy.

Were I to sit down and chart the serious bouts of depression and burnout I've navigated over the years, the one thing I am certain they would all have in common is that each episode occurred when I had wandered far from the creative path. Time and time again I have found myself falling into the deepest abyss when I have abandoned my creative soul and allowed other things to consume my time and my energy. Creativity is my lifeblood, and I have reached a point in my life where creative practice or expression has become an absolute non-negotiable for me. Just 15 minutes with felt tip pens and a colouring book offers much-needed respite from the hurricane that otherwise rages incessantly in my brain. It is the sweetest relief and essential in helping me manage ADHD without medication.

There is a mystical energy to creativity; something otherworldly about the brilliance that emerges when human beings conspire with this energy. However, I honestly believe that it's an energy

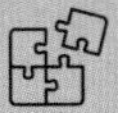

we are all entitled to and capable of harnessing. It doesn't have to be complicated. It doesn't have to be costly. You are under no pressure or obligation whatsoever to create something that will be admired or understood by anyone else but you.

Your practice can be a deeply personal affair that involves just you and inspiration; the ideation, exploration, and the making are their own reward, the result almost irrelevant. Or you might choose to share what you've made with the world because it allows you to make a statement about who you are and what matters to you, or because you simply love bringing joy and comfort to others with your unique ability to arrange colour or words or musical notes in a way that delights and soothes their soul as much as it does yours.

A joyful creative practice expects nothing of you. It makes no demands, and it has no agenda. It simply asks that you show up as often as you can and agree to collaborate with inspiration and whatever else drops into the space on any given day. Write, paint, sculpt, dance, sing, knit, sew, crochet, colour by numbers, plant a garden – do whatever you feel called to do and whatever gives you peace. Your heart and your soul will thank you for your commitment – as will your beautiful, if somewhat frazzled, brain.

SCAFFOLDING TO BUILD YOU UP

Channel your creativity

Creativity is within us all. Sometimes it's harder to reach for than others, but it's always there and it's our job to get quiet, listen, feel our intuitive hunches, and discover how we enjoy expressing our unique creativity.

Visualisation

Starting a creative pursuit might feel daunting if you have ADHD. But doing something creative and mindful doesn't have to require a huge amount of innate talent, expertise, or planning. It can be as simple as visualising something positive or enjoyable, such as a beach walk on a sunny day, taking a few minutes to brainstorm a new hobby or business idea, or thinking through creating positive lifestyle habits. Neuroscientific research strongly supports the benefits of using visualisation to welcome in powerful new ways of enjoying our lives.[49]

Pottering

Pottering is one of the greatest ways to kickstart creativity and leads to the ultimate feeling of being present. Pottering can look different for everyone, but it is generally considered to be the act of removing an outcome or the pressure for an activity to be productive. So, as ADHD people tend to be more restless internally and externally, pottering (which eliminates the need for a sense of achievement) is calming.

A favourite pottering pastime for me is to turn on the radio, make coffee, and potter in my kitchen without anyone else around. But pottering can involve any activity, such as cooking, gardening, folding the washing (if that's your bag!), or even decluttering. The caveat is that we must be alone to enjoy the

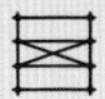

When we can channel our creativity we give ourselves permission to authentically show up as we are.

power of the pottering moment. This means we don't have to explain ourselves to anyone and can allow our brains to roam free. Think of it as being a free-range ADHD person in their natural habitat, with no rules and no pressure.

The key is to remove the expectation of productivity and do what you feel like doing (if anything) according to your energy levels. Spending alone time pottering helps me quieten my internal command sergeant who likes to bark instructions at me to be busy. I'm learning to hush this voice and become more open to the gentle whispers of 'process over purpose'.

Step away from distractions

You may feel you're too busy for creativity, or that as an adult you need to prioritise more important areas in your life such as work, finances, family, or ongoing responsibilities to others. With ADHD, many of us can relate to desperately clawing back time, working late into the night, or staying up too late to finally relax. But when you witness the incremental changes that follow from welcoming and making space for creativity in your life, you will know that it can impact your wellbeing in all areas.

You may have had a mindset that creativity is yet another job you might fail at or won't tick off the to-do list. But I promise that these pockets of creative moments will enhance your life beyond words and will impact you in ways that bring more rest, contentment, joy, mindfulness, hope, and fulfilment.
By exploring creativity we can step away from the mindless scrolling on our phones, shopping for more things we don't need but are driven by misdirected dopamine to buy, and recharge our batteries, ready to welcome in new ways of seeing the world, with all its possibilities and adventures.

TOOLS TO HELP

Unlock creativity

We're going to explore some of the ways you can unlock your creativity, get those juices flowing, and release more joy, fulfilment, flow, and mindfulness back into your life.

Set yourself some creativity guidelines

When it comes to accessing creativity, I do have some 'rules' to follow. When anything new is growing, providing the right environment is essential, and we need to extend this thinking to ourselves as we set about installing fresh creative patterns. My guidance for welcoming in more mindful and intentional creativity, especially for our ADHD brains, is as follows.

Remove the pressure of a definitive outcome: make your mantra 'process over outcome'.

When you engage in a creative activity, remove your phone or watch and let time just flow.

Release any thoughts of how you might monetise your creative output; allow this to be for your pleasure alone.

Only do what lights you up: no shoulds, needs, or ought tos; find something where time slips away and you feel fully present.

Lean into the fun and joy, without judging, doubting, or questioning yourself; when the self-criticism shows up, observe it and let it drift away.

There will always be a 'crappy first draft' (whether it's on paper or in another form); remember this and keep going.

Creativity comes from a growth mindset: curiosity, fun, and a willingness to learn, make mistakes, and even fail.

Allow yourself to pivot, change, and get bored; we no longer need to adhere to a set of rules that don't align with us anymore.

Give yourself permission to go leftfield: you don't need to make any announcements or tell anyone what you're doing. Keep this to yourself for as long as you want. We've been led to believe that everything we do must be chronicled on social media or in a WhatsApp group. On the contrary, the more private you keep your creative flow, the more authentic it will become, without the fear of judgement or comparison.

Get curious and ask yourself questions

If you are thinking, 'but I honestly don't know how to express my creativity', or if you find it hard to know what you truly enjoy, ask yourself these questions:

What are you naturally drawn to when looking at magazines? What is your current social media algorithm showing you? Let the things that genuinely interest you guide you without putting too much pressure on where it will take you.

What do you get excited about if it is randomly brought up in conversation?

Who would you love to ask many questions if you met them at a party or someone's house?

What do you notice about your thoughts when you are creative, compared to when you are worrying about the future or ruminating about the past?

How does your body feel when doing something you enjoy?

What emotions are bubbling up when you're so present and in the flow of the moment?

What leaves you feeling full, energised, and excited? Notice your body signs. Remember that energy, dopamine levels, and interest can ebb and flow, and it's okay to sometimes not feel like doing the thing you creatively enjoy.

Process and release the past through journalling

Externalising our thoughts through writing helps us to release stuck, negative emotions and process the confusing things our minds are struggling with, freeing us up for more creativity.

The Artist's Way by Julia Cameron is an inspirational guide for anyone who wants to develop more creative practices. One key takeaway is to create a 'morning pages' journal, which involves journalling whatever is on your mind to make space for more inspired thoughts. Using the prompts below as a starting point, try building this practice into your daily routine to help you tune into your mind and body and release what's keeping you stuck.

Morning pages journal prompts

Prompt 1...

What am I feeling in my body this morning?

Prompt 2...

Is there something intentional I'd like to achieve today?

Prompt 3...

Where can I lean into more joy and connection today?

Prompt 4...

What am I ready to let go of or release today?

Prompt 5...

How can I offer myself some love and self-compassion today?

Prompt 6...

Who can I reach out to and connect with today?

Be mindfully present

Making time to be creative can feel like an indulgence, but it has a crucial role in boosting wellbeing and mental health, and in rewiring neural pathways. Creativity also helps to reduce stress and increase feelings of fulfilment, connection, gratitude, and happiness. Try the following activities to help you to be more mindfully present.

- Walk or run in nature and listen to the sounds around you; notice what you can see and what has changed since your last visit to the same place.
- Play at spotting number signs on registration plates or houses.
- Practise EFT tapping, an incredible resource for grounding and keeping you in your body (see pp.42–43).
- Cook as a way to decompress and relax; some can find this stressful, as I do with baking, so just go with what keeps you mindful and in the moment.
- Spend time outside in nature: gardening, picking wild flowers, weeding, grounding your feet on the grass, and generally being aware of all the sensations around you.
- Try open water swimming or cold-water therapy in the bath or shower (see p.86). Research supports that just a few minutes in cold water achieves a 250% increase in dopamine and more than 500% boost in norepinephrine.[50]
- Focus on your breath and use techniques to keep you in the moment. Try box breathing (see p.60), or visualising the infinity sign (∞) to follow the in and out of your breath.

Strategies to take forward

Taking time to find this flow isn't selfish or wasteful – it's essential for your health and growth. Tuning in to creativity encourages moments of healing and connection and allows the mind to positively wander, telling your imagination it is safe to explore.

- Even on tricky days try to make time for mindful creativity and wellbeing practices such as journalling as a way to unblock your mind.
- Know that creativity can vary and is not prescriptive: it can include anything from gardening to singing.
- Allow yourself to feel curiosity and enthusiasm for trying new things. Let go, and don't be held back by the self-criticism of not being good enough or perceived failures in your past.
- Remember that pockets of sustained creativity and happiness are only possible when the mind and body are aligned, so prioritise your physical wellbeing too: hydrate, move your body, take time outside, and sleep and eat well.

REFLECTIVE MOMENT

What would you do creatively if you removed the idea of making money from it, the strategy, the cost, the qualifications, the comparison, the judgement, and the fear? If all those factors were removed, where do you see yourself getting creatively curious?

Write down whatever comes to mind and let it flow. Once it's out of your system, begin asking yourself what simple steps you could take to welcome this creative endeavour into your life right now. Remove any pressure or expectation – this is about curiosity without commitment.

CHAPTER 9

Lean Into Joy and Find Fulfilment

We're now going to talk about joy: this is something most of us give little or no conscious thought to, but it underpins our happiness and our sense of wellbeing. We'll explore its link to fulfilment, look at why so many of us with ADHD struggle to find it, and how to ensure that we do.

THE PROBLEM

When joy feels out of reach

Joy isn't problematic to define, yet for those of us with ADHD, it can be tricky to find. But what is joy?

According to the Oxford English Dictionary, it's 'a vivid emotion of pleasure arising from a sense of wellbeing or satisfaction'. I'm presuming this is not something many of us can relate to very often.

For those of us with ADHD, our default states are more often panic, dread, fear, worry, or hypervigilance. You'll no doubt know how easy it is to lose yourself in a spiral of 'have I done enough' worries, never-ending to-do lists, feelings of being unproductive, and 'what if' catastrophising – all creating anxiety, shame, and hypervigilance. This, in turn, can strengthen the neural pathways that lead to more repetitive negative thought cycles.

Though many of us will have developed anxious thought patterns, the neuroplasticity of our brains means we can also rewire our neural networks to help us experience more joy.

REWIRING THE BRAIN

The neuropsychologist Donald Hebb said in 1949, 'neurons that wire together, fire together'[51] – meaning that the more we do something, the stronger the neural networks become, making the practice easier each time. Tony Robbins, the motivational speaker and author, has said: 'Where focus goes, energy flows. And where energy flows, whatever you're focusing on grows. In other words, your life is controlled by what you focus on. That's why you need to focus on where you want to go, not on what you fear.'[52]

BREAKING IT DOWN

What's stopping us?

So, how do we find that elusive joy when our minds are often preoccupied with worries and 'what-ifs'?

The gift of gratitude

Gratitude is a perfect way to start your journey towards joy and increase your sense of fulfilment day by day. Instead of dwelling on the negative or fear-based thoughts in a situation, we can (as tricky as it may initially feel) actively explore a sense of gratitude to create more robust and positive neural pathways. This means that each time we seek out something to be thankful for, it becomes easier and more accessible. It takes time to proactively retrain our brains to seek the positives and then be grateful for even the most minor things, but we will slowly rewire the neurons in our brains to deliver more self-compassionate and positive thinking, leading to moments of intentional joy.

I was once guided by a deeply spiritual teacher who said that, if we're in doubt and lacking in clarity with what we want out of life, when we don't even know what to ask for in prayer or meditation, repeat the words 'Thank you. Thank you. Thank you' over and over. The energy of gratitude is powerful enough to move us from a place of worry and will enable us to find the good in even the direst of situations. The frequency of gratitude allows us to discover new possibilities and become open to fresh opportunities by building on what we already have. For example, if you're grateful for your deep friendships, then enhance these even more by reaching out and making plans with the people who lift you up. Or perhaps you can make new friends who are in a space you admire.

A joyful life is about the accumulation of tiny, wondrous moments and feeling a deep gratitude for them.

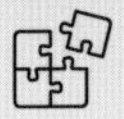

For me, joy doesn't have to be something monumental: it can be a morning coffee with the first rays of spring sun on my face; it can be a dog walk where there is finally no mud; or listening to a brand-new podcast featuring a favourite guest.

A morning cuddle with my youngest child elicits so much joy for me, it can carry me through the day. And yet, if I'm on my phone, checking social media and worrying about the time, I wouldn't be present enough to feel the joy of this beautiful moment that becomes so rare as our children grow older. But, as we're about to discover, gratitude isn't the only tool at our disposal.

The power of the present

I've taught myself, through lots of self-development work, that learning what I can control right now – as opposed to in five hours, days, weeks, or years – helps me feel calmer and happier. As simple as it sounds, I've also realised that I can only control what is *within* my control. I've always been drawn to pragmatic and clear-cut Stoic philosophy, the belief that we feel more joy if we focus our attention and energy on what we can control; it's a powerful antidote to the ADHD tendency to feel anxious about the future.

Understanding this sphere of control will become an important part of our toolkit for cultivating joy (see p.166), but we must first learn to recognise the times when we feel out of control.

WHAT'S WITHIN YOUR CONTROL

Stoic thinking (which focuses on what you can control in the present as a way of overcoming negative thoughts) has been developed by the positive psychology movement into the circle of control theory, adding a 'sphere of influence' into the mix: a grey zone between what we can and cannot control.

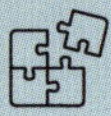

Positive psychology and ADHD

RUTH KUDZI, master certified coach, coaching psychologist, consultant, and trainer

“*Integrate positive psychology tools such as gratitude into your daily practice. When we practise gratitude, we strengthen neural pathways and release dopamine, so we are increasing our propensity to experience positive emotions, which in turn helps enhance wellbeing. You can start with a daily practice, either in the morning or evening, when you reflect on three things that you're grateful for and take time sitting with those feelings.*

Strengths-based approaches can also be beneficial to build confidence when you have ADHD. We can feel like we're in a deficit model focused on what we're not good at, but by reframing and looking at what you're good at and working on these characteristics, you can flourish. For example, my creativity is a super strength, and I spend time working on it rather than looking at my lack of organisation or follow-through. You can identify your strengths through personal reflection, using specific tools, asking up to 10 close friends/co-workers/acquaintances who know you well for three strengths they see in you, or working with a coach.

Another powerful tool is visualisation (see p.148): spending time connecting with who you want to become and what you want to achieve can enhance your positive emotions and wellbeing. This is not always accessible to everyone with ADHD, as some people are unable to visualise. If this is you, vision boards can be another tool that can help you value tag what is important and motivate you to pursue your goals.

Finally, consider how you're building and maintaining your relationships, as often there is a co-occurrence of rejection sensitive disorder (see pp.46–63) with ADHD that can make it challenging. Focusing on positive interactions with others and filling your inner circle with those that you trust can help you increase wellbeing and feel less isolated. You might seek out others in the community to strengthen your network and sense of belonging too.”

SCAFFOLDING TO BUILD YOU UP

The journey to joy

Joy and fulfilment are closer than you think. By making a few simple changes to your everyday life, you can move one step closer to experiencing them.

Protect your energy

Fulfilment is messy and imperfect. Finding it doesn't mean we have to give all of ourselves to other people and situations; on the contrary, it means we need to instil firm boundaries, respect our energy reserves, and honour what makes us tick. We have to build an energetic fortress around ourselves, because when we find fulfilment in helping and serving others, our resources and reserves are paramount: we can't pour from an empty cup. We don't keep our mobile at 5% battery – the low-battery mode is there for a reason, telling us it can be used for emergencies only. To find fulfilment and cultivate joy we have to nurture and conserve our energy to be the person we want to show up as.

Live by your values

As our priorities and values change and evolve, so do the things that fulfil us. I noticed this when I had been coaching for a while, and I wanted the opportunity to learn and grow while also helping more people. This came through launching my first podcast, The Ambitious Mum, which tapped into my core values, including creativity, curiosity, expansion, fun, growth, learning, and connection. Looking inwards and identifying your core values *(see p.168)* will help you make life choices that build on these, bringing you closer to fulfilment.

IN HER SHOES

I'm a great encourager, because I always see the potential in others. What helps me feel more fulfilled is teaching, learning something new, and spending time with family.

Leigh, 58

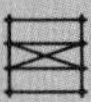

Embrace your magnetic desires

With ADHD, we tend to have a lot of 'magnetic desires', or what is sometimes called 'shiny object syndrome'. We often like to take up exciting hobbies, before getting bored and moving on to the next dopamine-delivering activity. This is not something to feel ashamed of. In fact, the most successful ADHD people I know bank all the wisdom, experience, and insights they've gained from having multiple interests, hobbies, or careers and use them to seek valuable opportunities. The more skills and knowledge we have, the more we can unlock our purpose and find satisfaction in our achievements.

Understand your purpose

Even when we are practising gratitude, a lack of purpose in what we are doing will ultimately lead us to feeling unfulfilled. It is important that we stop for long enough to recognise where we are feeling discontented in order to make positive changes.

In around 2012 I started feeling an intense desire to accomplish something outside of my family dynamic but was overwhelmed by my many commitments. When I look back at that version of me, I see a woman brimming with ideas, desperately trying to fulfil her creativity and make a difference in other people's lives.

I decided to retrain as a health coach, and as I built up my skill set, I noticed how my yearning for fulfilment was abating. What kept driving me through all the difficult moments of self-doubt, confusion, imposter syndrome, and fear was the feeling of delight in my achievements. I noticed the joyous high I'd get after a session with a client who told me that an emotion or long-standing belief had shifted or been released.

When I discovered my ADHD, I knew that this was not only the missing piece in my life, but also in so many of my clients' lives. Finally, I had the answers I had deeply craved, and I was ready to reframe the narrative I had been feeding myself for so long.

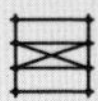

Fulfilment

SARI SOLDEN, author, ADHD expert, therapist, and consultant

" *No one usually asks the critical question about how women with ADHD, especially after a late diagnosis, can move towards fulfilment. Instead, they usually ask about how to become organised, how to be on time, how to be like other people, or how to get everything done.*

In reality, a life of meaning, authenticity, connection, and self-acceptance adds up to fulfilment. The important steps that often follow a diagnosis – such as medication, understanding, support, and strategies for executive function challenges – must all be in the service of leading a fulfilling life, not only to be organised for its own sake or as a measure of your own worth.

The goal after a diagnosis for a woman with ADHD is to move towards a compelling vision of the future. This will help not only with activating her brain, but will also activate the process of healing. In other words, the key to fulfilment is to be driven not only by the goal of reduction of symptoms, but also by moving towards a values-driven life – to see herself as a whole woman including her strengths, struggles, and a firm core sense of self. To do this requires healing the wounds that have been acquired as a result of not understanding confusing developmental experiences for such a large portion of her life. It requires repair of a self-image that has often been understandably distorted by years of not understanding all of who she is.

Fulfilment for a woman with ADHD after an adult diagnosis comes as a result of forming connections where she is seen and valued. It comes from creating a life where she does not hide in shame or a life where she tries to just fit in, but instead one in which she moves towards a life of purpose, free to use her voice, and to ask for the support she needs in order to make her unique contribution to the world. "

TOOLS TO HELP

Manifest joy

Here are some practical tools to help you move away from worry and fear and begin experiencing more joy in your daily life.

Understand your sphere of influence

Earlier in this chapter, we discussed the Stoic concept of the spheres of control (see p.161), which psychologists have expanded to include a sphere of influence. Often, fears, worries, or anxieties beyond our control can get in the way of our ability to experience joy. By recognising that we cannot change the things outside of our control and focusing our energy on what we can influence, we can bring ourselves closer to experiencing joy.

What does your sphere of influence look like? Take a moment to write down all of the fears, worries, or anxieties that get in the way of you experiencing joy. Now categorise these into things within your circle of control or influence, and things you cannot control.

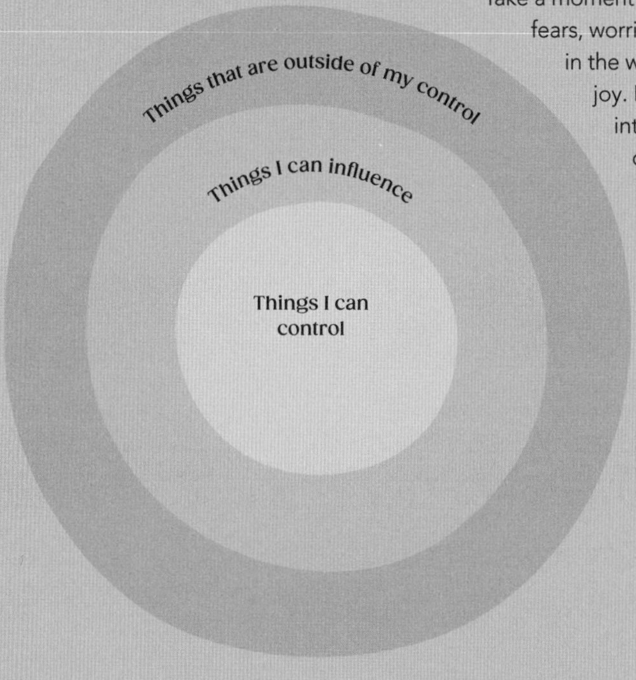

Things that are outside of my control

Things I can influence

Things I can control

Value tagging and manifesting

Dr Tara Swart is a neuroscientist and author of *The Source*, a book about manifesting our magnetic desires. She talks about the notion of 'value tagging' to help turn our desires into reality. By visually depicting our desires in an action or vision board, we are telling our brains what to aim for and focus on. We are kickstarting the Reticular Activating System (RAS), the part of the brain that highlights and detects what we're focusing on.

We may think it's coincidental that when we want to book a holiday to Italy, suddenly every magazine features articles on Italian getaways; this is our brain homing in on what we want and helping us sieve out the dross to be more targeted with our desires. This is why creating a vision board that aligns with our brain's wiring works so well. Dr Swart's work has helped to marry the concept of manifestation with science, leading to manifesting being endorsed by the neuroscience community.

Creating a vision board

1. ***Think about how you like to visualise***
   This might be words, drawings, or photographs.

2. ***Reflect on your desires***
   Scribble them down to reduce the overwhelm.

3. ***Gather materials***
   Collect sources that represent your vision.

4. ***Create your board***
   Scatter it with words, drawings, images, or flow charts.

5. ***Have fun with it***
   Allow your vision board to develop and change as you grow.

Identify your core values

A powerful way to discover fulfilment is by identifying your core values and understanding that these are the drivers making you tick. If they aren't being met, there is a high chance your foundations will feel rocky and inauthentic. A simple exercise is to list 15–20 core values (see examples opposite), such as honesty, connection, creativity, justice, and growth. Try not to overthink these, and write them as they come to you. Once you have your list, choose the five that resonate the most right now, and use these to steer you when making important choices about your life. Ask yourself:

- Which of your five core values are currently being met and which aren't?
- If the values are being met, but feel minimised, what steps can you take to help them play a more prominent role?
- What is preventing any core values that aren't being addressed from being met in your daily life?

Identifying the root cause of feeling frustrated, intolerant, impatient, or resentful about life right now allows us to recognise where more clarity and new boundaries may be needed. For example, if your creativity and connection values aren't being addressed and they could increase your sense of fulfilment, have you checked out local art clubs or workshops?

Authenticity

Achievement

Adventure

Beauty

Balance

Compassion

Challenge

Competency

Creativity

Community

Fairness

Faith

Contribution

Determination

Honesty

Growth

Trust

Humour

Openness

Kindness

Self-respect

Fun

Wisdom

Wealth

Stability

Peace

Speak openly about your ADHD

You may have noticed that when you either gained your diagnosis or simply became aware of ADHD, the mask slipped away and more of your ADHD traits came to the fore. Perhaps you felt safer to be open with your trusted family and friends, allowing you to 'out' your ADHD when something more challenging came up. When you feel secure enough to share your ADHD, you are able to live life with more honesty.

Practise gratitude

Practising gratitude can help you notice the things in your life that already bring you a feeling of purpose and contentment. Perhaps you're not feeling satisfied at work right now but have a beautiful group of close friends you feel connected to. Could you be grateful that you have fulfilment in your social life and accept that your career is not your focus right now? Feeling fulfilled simply means that something you're doing right now is filling your cup; your soul's desires are being met in some capacity, and it's okay to not have all your life figured out.

REFLECTIVE MOMENT

Jot down the things that you are grateful for right now. Don't overthink it, your first ideas are fine – it can be anything from that hot cup of coffee in front of you to gratitude for support from a close friend. How does reflecting on these things, even briefly, make you feel?

Strategies to take forward

Joyfulness is a wonderful, life-enhancing state and I want you all to experience it. You deserve it and all the happiness and contentment it will bring. These final thoughts will help guide you towards a place of fulfilment.

- Take time to identify your core values and then actively and intentionally seek new ways to incorporate them into your daily life, career, family, and relationships.
- Recognise the small activities that fill you with joy and hope, the people who light you up, and the meaningful everyday touchstones that allow you to find more moments of joy.
- Visual reminders are a great help. Print out a 'joy list' and keep it somewhere you can see it every day. This gentle nudge may be all you need to make more intentional choices in your daily life and not have to wait for that holiday or day off in order to seek joy; a micro-moment of joy every day has more of a positive and incremental impact.
- Be open to growth and new opportunities, and recognise that life is forever an unfinished project, that we have choices to keep growing and evolving and it's okay to make mistakes.

REFLECTIVE MOMENT

Nature brings me a huge amount of joy: breathing in fresh air, taking in greenery, and simply moving my body outside are my ways of processing. I know this isn't possible for everyone, but try to identify a place that fills you with joy, which is accessible and free. When we find joy in these simple places, we can fire up our neurons to more easily identify other ways of seeking daily joy, such as a cuddle with our dog, a baby's giggle, a phone call with a friend – it's really up to you.

CHAPTER 10

Simplify Life

We're nearly at the end of our journey together, although I'll emphasise again that the process of moving towards calm, acceptance, and fulfilment isn't linear. In this final chapter, we'll talk about simplifying life so that, despite the external challenges you might face, you can work towards feeling a greater sense of inner peace and self-acceptance.

THE PROBLEM

Our inner battle

As we've explored throughout the book, our overworked dopamine-seeking ADHD brains desperately crave regulation and calm, yet we struggle to access this naturally.

If you are living with ADHD, you can probably relate to the internalised noise and chaos that can cause you to feel depleted, drained of energy, and out of control. Our neurodivergent brain structure, wiring, hormones, and chemical make-up mean we face challenges around focus, impulsivity, planning, time management, prioritising, motivation, execution, and memory. So no matter how much we crave structure, calm, and simplicity, we can struggle to achieve it without extra help and support.

One of the most powerful tools to help us navigate ADHD is to intentionally strip back and simplify life wherever we can. This can be through our homes, our many ADHD-curated systems, how we want to work, and the way we live. I often live by the following mantra: how can I simplify this situation to reduce the feeling of being overwhelmed and anxious?

Simplifying life by being open to new ways of living, working, and parenting can all be done if we're willing to think beyond what we've been conditioned to believe is the 'right' way of doing things. By getting curious about the unrealistic standards we may have set ourselves and unlearning what we've been told, we can offload much of the baggage that has been slowing us down. A powerful way to harness our newly acquired perspective is to actively lower the perfectionist expectations and demands we place upon ourselves.

IN HER SHOES

Pre-diagnosis? In a nutshell, life was chaotic, and I was constantly overwhelmed. Being perimenopausal didn't help. I was always wondering when I would figure out how to be organised. To outsiders, they think I'm one of the most organised people!

Tanya, 49

BREAKING IT DOWN

Why we struggle

We're now going to examine some of the ways in which ADHD can work against us, making it hard for us to introduce (and stick to) the changes that we need to make in order to simplify life.

The daily struggle

Recognising our challenges with executive functioning is key to understanding why simplifying life often feels so hard to achieve. We can struggle to sustain focus, prioritise and finish tasks, make decisions, and maintain a routine. We also often have working memory challenges, meaning we can miss important things and dates. All of this can make navigating life in a neurotypical world exhausting and chaotic. Once we recognise and lean into these differences with self-compassion, we can begin living in a way that feels calmer, more effortless, and a little simpler.

The dopamine rollercoaster

The connection between the 'feel-good' hormone dopamine and ADHD is well known; we can be deficient in dopamine or struggle to regulate it. This can contribute to many challenging features of ADHD such as low mood, addictive behaviours, impulsivity, irritability, lack of focus, and poor motivation.[53] If you are living with ADHD you might be familiar with the 'dopamine push and pull' – a mood and energy rollercoaster that often feels out of control. Some days we are flooded with dopamine, so we might overcommit. Then, only 24 hours later, comes the dreaded energy ebb; our dopamine levels dip, contributing to a low mood and lack of desire to commit to the plans we previously made.[54] This habit of saying yes to things we lack the time, energy, or mental headspace for can lead to chaos and overwhelm. Recognising the dopamine-driven highs and lows is the first step towards simplifying life.

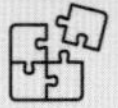

Managing dopamine

NICOLE VIGNOLA, neuroscientist, author, and keynote speaker

“ *Dopamine is not the only neurochemical at play in ADHD, but it's one of the major driving forces. For example, dopamine helps us to accurately judge the passing of time; dysfunction in the dopamine system can lead to either underestimating the time that something would take or overestimating it. Think about when you're having a good time and it feels as though it goes by really quickly – it's because your dopamine levels are really high. This is one of the reasons why ADHDers might find themselves not having good time management.*

Also, dopamine is a reward-based learning activity. You know the feeling when you do something right and have a 'yes, tick, I feel good about myself' moment? This releases dopamine, and the positive reinforcement has a cumulative, snowball effect. We need to choose our activities wisely.

One of my biggest hacks is trying not to be on my phone for the first hour of the morning, because that really jacks up dopamine levels. The problem with this is that it sets the trajectory of reward-seeking behaviour for the rest of the day, and it means by three o clock I'm like a junkie scrolling social media. It's one of the hardest habits to break, though.

The other side of this is limiting phone use late at night. Research shows that after 11pm screen usage affects the way that we create dopamine because it impacts an area of the brain called the habenula. The habenula regulates dopamine activity overnight, and exposure to artificial light during times when your circadian rhythm signals sleep disrupts this process. This interference suppresses dopamine production, leading to lower dopamine levels overnight, which can negatively impact mood and motivation. It is important to work with your body to keep your dopamine levels regulated; if you do you will feel the impact in many areas of your life. ”

SCAFFOLDING TO BUILD YOU UP

How to simplify life

So, what simple steps can we take to make life feel more manageable and to soothe our minds? Here are my top strategies for simplifying life.

Declutter your mind and physical space

I have found living with less stuff and gaining more control and responsibility over my belongings life changing. Decluttering your space is not only hugely regulating and therapeutic for the mind, but it can calm the soul too. It comes back to the need for simplification, reducing sensory overload.

One way to stop accumulating more possessions is to concentrate on trading stuff for memories. Worldly possessions are less important than connections, loving moments, and memories. Focusing on our relationships can replace the dopamine we used to get from shopping and scrolling. Noticing how we unhealthily seek dopamine is the first step, and then we can begin replacing it with healthier strategies for obtaining a happiness buzz.

Think about people and situations

Simplifying life doesn't just require looking at our external surroundings; we can take an inventory of people and situations that cause us to feel anxious and on edge. Now we see ADHD for what it is, we get to question the decisions and choices we make with more integrity and deeper understanding.

Step outside of yourself and do some intentional digging to see what's going on. Think about the ways you are complicating your life. Perhaps you are adding unnecessary work to the load, saying yes too much, or putting all of your self-worth into being productive. Are you taking on more to gain the external validation you never received as a child? Are you people-pleasing without any boundaries to feel accepted? Are you signing up for more courses to prove something to yourself and others? What is

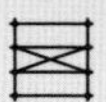

the deeper reason for wanting this ongoing busyness and noise in your life, and what's stopping you from finding fulfilment, satisfaction, and contentment in calmer and less chaotic ways? You may not be ready to pull back from all the 'extra' areas of your life – they will often be bringing you joy and fun as well as overwhelm. But just recognising the consequences of what you're taking on may help you make a more aligned decision next time you crave adding an extra layer of 'clutter' to your life.

Learning to rest

I used to want to fill my life with different businesses, hobbies, arrangements, and people. I thought I had to keep up with my busy ideas, and all of them had to be implemented. Yet my nervous system and energy levels were crying out for rest. Part of simplifying my life has been moving away from 'doing' and leaning more into 'being'. The more I understand the neurodivergent community, the more I realise that we should be less like worker bees and more like lionesses, resting and recharging to ensure that when we need energy surges for the big and important work, we have enough in reserve. Resting is not weak; with rest, we can receive incredible downloads of ideas and intuition. In these moments of downtime I have my greatest flashes of inspiration. Rest is my greatest asset, and it can be yours, too. We must reprogramme how we see rest and look at it as the most productive part of our day.

REFLECTIVE MOMENT

Think of a time where you felt drained and exhausted by what you added to your plate without awareness. What was the lead up to this? Could you cope?

Now, think of a time when you felt empowered and strong enough to say no. How did it feel, and what contributed to it? I expect, at least in part, you felt relieved and grateful.

Use this data to help inform future decision-making moments.

TOOLS TO HELP

Keep it simple

Here are some practical suggestions for simplifying your world and moving from chaos to calm, both now and in the future.

SIMPLIFY YOUR...	HOW?
Cooking and shopping	• Try online shopping and keep a virtual shopping basket of ingredients you always need. • Keep an active shopping list on your phone or on the fridge, as well as quick recipe ideas that are nutritious, reflect what people in the house like, and don't take too much time. • Discard those long recipes with far too many ingredients and find a simpler option, or create your own version instead. • Meal prep boxes, pre-chopped or frozen vegetables, and healthy convenience food such as fresh soups or sauces.
Work	• Find the time, space, and routines where your best self is allowed to thrive. Now that more companies understand the importance of diversity, equality, and inclusion (DEI), neurodivergent needs are slowly being met. • Lengthy business systems or too many unnecessary meetings discussing the same thing over and over? Propose some more neurodivergent-friendly options such as walking meetings, flexible working hours, and allowing things like headphones and fidget toys.

SIMPLIFY YOUR...	HOW?
Routine	• Consider the night before what might make your morning easier and then work towards creating a morning routine that's simple, effective, and fast. • Block out pockets of undisturbed rest in your diary such as meditative practices, calming, mindful movement, or time in nature. • Track your burnout signs and pull back from commitments when they appear. • Prioritise simple self-care: an early night, stretching, time with friends, hobbies, or time off. • Research low-demand parenting options that help you reduce the ongoing societal pressures, demands, and expectations of neurodivergent parenting.
Finances	• Download neurodivergent-friendly bank apps, such as Monzo; these recognise our different struggles with money, and help us keep tabs with simple and well-mapped graphics and systems. • Evaluate behaviours that are leading you into financial difficulty. For example, deactivate a credit card or fast-payment accounts, remove shopping apps from your phone, and unsubscribe from tempting newsletters. • Put some basic parameters in place: allow yourself a 10-minute window per day or week to scroll websites of shops that you love but stick to the limits you set.

SIMPLIFY YOUR...	HOW?
Friendships and relationships	• Connect with like-minded people and begin to distance yourself from inauthentic friendships or activities. Say 'no more' to what you want to release in your life, such as toxic friendships or demanding relationships, and 'yes' to fewer people. Be more mindful of the yeses: make sure they are the 'hell yeses', and if they aren't, practise politely declining for now. • Leave WhatsApp groups that are draining and time-consuming and ask a reliable friend to notify you if something pressing comes up. • Keep a daily boundaries check-in to help you identify with whom, how, and when they are compromised, allowing you to recognise the signs earlier. Once we get comfortable with asserting our boundaries it becomes second nature and is no longer a difficult conversation.
House	• Once a week, commit to removing one or two items from the house. Incremental micro-moments of decluttering are easy to cope with and remove the overwhelm of a weekend of energy-depleting skip-filling.
Options	• Intentionally look for the simplest option in every decision. This could be taking hand luggage only when travelling, stripping back social plans, or removing complicated systems at work.

SIMPLIFY YOUR...	HOW?
Mind	• Take some time to feel present every day, this could be a phone-free walk, car journey listening to relaxing music, or a yoga class. • Writing out our busy thoughts also helps externalise the chaos and welcomes in the calm we seek. • Try a few minutes of tapping each day to help declutter your busy mind, regain perspective, and process and release any stuck emotions.
Time	• Recognise that time is your most precious commodity. Weigh up what you can let go of to create more space and time in your life for moments of presence. • Become more mindful of what you commit to and pause before you say yes to anything. • Spend five minutes a day unsubscribing from accounts and emails that eat into your precious time. • Put your phone out of sight to spend more time being present with loved ones. • Replace time-draining habits with activities you genuinely enjoy. For example, if the gym feels like a chore, consider joining a climbing club or taking up another hobby that brings you more joy and motivation.

Take the simplest option

Think about how you can adopt a simpler approach in every area of life. Using the below examples as guidance, pick a scenario from your own life and create a 'try this' option for next time?

INSTEAD OF THIS		TRY THIS
Overwhelming, noisy WhatsApp group chats, trying to sort out big-group arrangements with complicated logistics.	→	Message friends directly and arrange to meet them one-on-one at a time and place that feels good to you.
Deciding to declutter your *entire* house or wardrobe in one day.	→	Choose one small area to work on at a time, keeping a charity bag close to hand, enabling you to do manageable microbursts of organising.
Worrying about forgetting important dates or anniversaries and the gift-buying that's needed.	→	Set aside a morning, put all of the dates you don't want to miss in your online diary, with reminders and links to e-gift vouchers.
Feeling like you have to join a gym to exercise.	→	Discover fun ways to move your body that work for you, such as trampolining, skating, boxing, or dog walking.
Thinking you need to plan for special family days out.	→	Choose to be okay with activities around the house, such as crafts, baking, gardening, or painting a fence.

Strategies to take forward

Simplifying your life sounds like it should be easy, and yet, courtesy of our restless, dopamine-seeking brains, it can feel anything but. But the benefits of introducing some changes that keep your life calmer – whether that's from a sensory point of view, a practical or an emotional one – are huge. Here are my final thoughts on how you can take some steps towards achieving a feeling of peace and expansiveness.

- Recognise the power of stillness and silence to create a tranquil environment that is yours alone.
- Give yourself permission to create a sacred space that provides you with a calming sanctuary, whether that's a clean car, kitchen, or a bathroom with essential oils and bath salts.
- Surround yourself with people, objects, and energy that uplift, empower, and ground you: tell yourself that you deserve the absolute best.
- Recognise that life is much too short to feel burnt out, depleted, and dysregulated, and look for times when you can prioritise yourself and choose to do things differently.

REFLECTIVE MOMENT

Let's take a moment to consider what changes you could make right now, or in the coming days, to help you achieve the goal of a more simplified life.

Can you choose three things you are ready to unsubscribe from today?

Is there one thing that feels like it's had an expiration date you've been ignoring?

Where are you being intuitively called to create more simplicity in your life?

Conclusion

Thank you for reading this book. I hope you've discovered tools to empower you on your ADHD journey; and don't be afraid to return to the relevant chapters when you need to lean into specific strategies and ideas. As we know, ADHD likes to bring all sorts of energy, moods, and emotions to the surface to keep us on our toes!

This book is not about eliminating ADHD symptoms and traits; that is nearly impossible. But I do hope that my guidance has brought you more clarity, inner peace, self-compassion, and – most importantly – self-awareness. Self-awareness is half the battle when it comes to improving life with ADHD and lessening the impact of the more challenging symptoms we've lived with for most of our lives. When we understand why we think, feel, and act the way we do, everything else becomes a lot easier.

If you've read this book as someone who was diagnosed later in life and has spent many decades feeling clueless about your brain's different wiring, I hope the information has been met with forgiveness and love for yourself and all that you haven't been aware of.

Understanding yourself

As you now know, ADHD can show up differently for everyone, and we are all faced with different circumstances in life. There may be times when your ADHD is a mere nuisance, and others where it is all-encompassing and debilitating – and that's okay. Please don't criticise yourself if you find life suddenly becomes unmanageable, or you feel like you are struggling to uphold the changes you have worked hard to make. The key is to recognise when you are struggling, send yourself some love, and ask yourself what you can do to get back on track. Just take one small step in the right direction, whether that's drinking a glass of water or going for a 10-minute walk. Make no judgement, allow no self-criticism, and just acknowledge that you're doing the best you can in your current circumstances. Undoing long-established patterns is hard, and even when those patterns have been difficult and traumatic, at least we've known what to expect. With new awareness and our eyes opened to other possibilities, it may cause relationships, jobs, friendships, lifestyles, and mindsets to be dismantled. It can be terrifying not knowing what will be rebuilt in their place, but ultimately this can be liberating, too.

Utilising your potential

You are now on a new and possibly unnerving path of self-understanding and discovery. My parting words are to trust yourself. Trust that you know what's best for you, and that you have it within you to make choices that work for your mind and body. Allow this new understanding of your wiring to be a gift and no longer a curse. Listen to your body's wisdom, and give it space to communicate with you. Begin to lean into expression and stop suppressing your emotions, desires, and needs.

Recognise that you are important and that asking for help and support is okay. Although you may have always been the one to care for others, forsaking your own dreams, allow this book to now care for you. Re-read it in a bath filled with essential oils or listen to the audio version while walking, whenever you need a reminder to value yourself; take time to heal, process, and relearn a new life on terms that work and uplift you, which empower and motivate you to feel like the best version of yourself. Recognise that you are deserving of all this, and be the person you yearned for all those years ago when you weren't shown the care, love, and support you needed and were worthy of.

Make time to pause, breathe, and visualise a new way of living that feels more effortless, simple, hopeful, and joyful, for that is what we all deserve. And, importantly, model this for all the generations ahead who are looking to us to pave a new road where women are listened to, heard, validated, supported, and celebrated in all our messy brilliance.

Endnotes

1. Susan Young, Nicoletta Adamo and Bryndis Björk Ásgeirsdóttir, et al., 'Females with ADHD', BMC Psychiatry, 20, 404, 2020

2. Stephen Hinshaw, Elizabeth Owens and Christine Zalecki, et al., 'Prospective follow-up of girls with attention-deficit/hyperactivity disorder into early adulthood', Journal of Consulting and Clinical Psychology, 13 Aug 2012, 80(6), pp. 1041–1051

3. IBS: Kedem S, Yust-Katz S, Carter D, Levi Z, Kedem R, Dickstein A, Daher S, Katz LH, 'Attention Deficit Hyperactivity Disorder and Gastrointestinal Morbidity in a Large Cohort of Young Adults', World J Gastroenterol, November 2020

Fibromyalgia: Ertan Yilmaz and Lut Tamam , 'Attention-deficit hyperactivity disorder and impulsivity in female patients with fibromyalgia', Neuropsychiatric Disease and Treatment, 2018, 14: pp. 1883–18890

Chronic Fatigue Syndrome: 'ADHD and Chronic Fatigue Syndrome: Understanding the Complex Relationship', NeuroLaunch online, August 2024

Adrenal fatigue: Pin-Han Peng, Meng-Yun Tsai and Sheng-Yu Lee, et al., 'Attention-Deficit/Hyperactivity Disorder, Its Pharmacotherapy, and Adrenal Gland Dysfunction', International Journal of Environmental Research and Public Health, 25 May 2020, 17(10): 3709

Chronic pain: Eleanor Battison, Patrick Brown, Amy Holley and Anna Wilson, 'Associations between Chronic Pain and Attention-Deficit Hyperactivity Disorder (ADHD) in Youth', 11 Jan 2023, 10(1): 142

Migraines: Thomas Hansen, Louise Hoeffding and Lisette Kogelman, et al., 'Comorbidity of migraine with ADHD in adults', BMC Neurology 18, 147, 2018

Autoimmune conditions: Tor-Arne Hegvik, Qi Chen and Ralf Kuja-Halkola, et al., 'Familial co-aggregation of attention-deficit/hyperactivity disorder and autoimmune diseases', International Journal of Epidemiology, vol. 51, Issue 3, June 2022, pp. 898–909

Postnatal depression and perinatal anxiety: Anneli Andersson, Miguel Garcia-Argibay and Alexander Victorin, et al., 'Depression and anxiety disorders during the postpartum period in women diagnosed with attention deficit hyperactivity disorder', Journal of Affective Disorders, vol. 325, 15 March 2023, pp. 817–823

ADHD and social anxiety: Ahmet Koyuncu, Erhan Ertekin and Çağri Yüksel, et al., 'Predominantly Inattentive Type of ADHD Is Associated With Social Anxiety Disorder', Journal of Attention Disorders, 19(10), 2015, pp. 856–864

4. SV Faraone and H Larsson, 'Genetics of attention deficit hyperactivity disorder', Molecular Psychiatry 24, 2019, pp. 562–575

5. Christian Jacob, Silke Gross-Lesch and Thomas Jans, et al., 'Internalizing and externalizing behavior in adult ADHD', ADHD Atten Def Hyp Disord, vol. 6, 2014, pp. 101–110

6. Isabel Schnorr, Anne Siegl and Sonja Luckhardt, et al., 'Inflammatory biotype of ADHD is linked to chronic stress', Translational Psychiatry, 14, 37 (2024)

7. Kelly Duffy, Keri Rosch and Mary Beth Nebel, et al., 'Increased integration between default mode and task-relevant networks in children with ADHD is associated with impaired response control', Developmental Cognitive Neuroscience, 22 June 2021, vol. 50:100980

8. ibid

9. Ellen Littman, PhD, 'Rejection Sensitivity Is Worse for Girls and Women with ADHD', Additude magazine, 5 June 2023, available at: www.additudemag.com/rejection-sensitivity-women-adhd/

10. Naomi Eisenberger, Matthew Lieberman and Kipling Williams, 'Does rejection hurt? An FMRI study of social exclusion', Science, 10 Oct 2003, 302(5643), pp. 290–2

11. Daniel G Amen and Blake D Carmichael, 'High-resolution brain SPECT imaging in ADHD', Annals of Clinical Psychiatry 9(2), 1 June 1997, pp. 81–6

12. Amy FT Arnsten, 'The Emerging Neurobiology of Attention Deficit Hyperactivity Disorder', The Journal of Pediatrics, 1 May 2009; 154(5):I-S43

13. Kazuhiro Tajima-Pozo, Miguel Yus and Gonzalo Ruiz-Manrique, et al., 'Amygdala Abnormalities in Adults With ADHD', Journal of Attention Disorders, vol. 22, 10 March 2016

14. Naomi P Friedman and Trevor W Robbins, 'The role of prefrontal cortex in cognitive control and executive function', Neuropsychopharmacology, vol. 47, 18 August 2021, pp. 72–89

15. Charlie Elizabeth Culverhouse, 'Kids with ADHD receive more "negative messages" than neurotypical kids', Good to Know magazine, 15 May 2024

16. Olivia Guy-Evans, MSc, 'Parasympathetic Nervous System (PSNS) Functions & Division', Simply Psychology, 21 Sept 2023

17. Nicole Brown, Suzette Brown and Rahil Briggs, et al., 'Associations Between Adverse Childhood Experiences and ADHD Diagnosis and Severity', Academic Pediatrics, vol. 17, 2017, pp. 349–355

18. 'What Happens to Your Nervous System While You Sleep', Flowly, n.d.

19. Tracy Otsuka, 'How to Break the Exhausting Habit of Revenge Bedtime Procrastination', Additude magazine, 11 June 2024

20. Chun Shen, Qiang Luo and Samuel R Chamberlain, et al., 'What Is the Link Between Attention-Deficit/Hyperactivity Disorder and Sleep Disturbance?', Biological Psychiatry, 15 Sept 2020, 88(6): pp. 459–469

21. Roberta D Brinton, Jia Yao and Fei Yin et al., 'Perimenopause as a neurological transition state', Nature

Reviews Endocrinology, 26 May 2015; 11(7), pp.393–405

Anne Caufriez, Rachel Leproult and Mireille L'Hermite-Balériaux, et al., 'Progesterone Prevents Sleep Disturbances and Modulates GH, TSH, and Melatonin Secretion in Postmenopausal Women', The Journal of Clinical Endocrinology & Metabolism, vol. 96, Issue 4, 1 April 2011

22. Nisha Charkoudian and Jennifer Rabbitts, 'Sympathetic nervous system and volume-regulatory hormones', Physiology News Magazine, winter 2010, Issue 81

23. Natalie Pross, Agnès Demazières and Nicolas Girard, et al., 'Effects of changes in water intake on mood of high and low drinkers', PLoS One, 11 April 2014

24. Amy Paturel, 'Bolster Your Brain by Stimulating the Vagus Nerve', Cedars Sinai blog, 21 March 2024

25. Marc Nornstein and Gianluca Esposito, 'Coregulation: A Multilevel Approach via Biology and Behavior', 31 July 2023, Children (Basel)

26. JS Kooij, 'Hormonal sensitivity of mood symptoms in women with ADHD across the lifespan', European Psychiatry, 19 July 2023

Bethan Roberts, Tory Eisenlohr-Moul and Michelle M Martel, 'Reproductive steroids and ADHD symptoms across the menstrual cycle', Psychoneuroendocrinology, 28 Nov 2018, pp. 105–114,

27. Anni Layne Rodgers, 'We Demand Attention on the Elevated Risk for PMDD and PPD Among Women with ADHD', Additude magazine, 21 May 2024

28. 'ADHD Impairment Peaks in Menopause, According to ADDitude Reader Survey', Additude magazine, 19 April 2024

29. Anni Layne Rodgers, 'We Demand Attention on the Elevated Risk for PMDD and PPD Among Women with ADHD', Additude magazine, 21 May 2024

30. Closing the Women's Health Gap, World Economic Forum and McKinsey Health Institute, Jan 2024

31. Benjamin Pollock, 'Downplayed distress: Gaslighting in women's healthcare', The Daily Free Press, 11 April 2023

32. Kate Whiting, 'Women's health gap: 6 conditions that highlight gender inequality in healthcare', World Economic Forum, 14 Oct 2024

33. 'Menopause: identification and management', NICE guidelines [NG23], 12 November 2015 (updated 7 November 2024)

34. 'ADHD Impairment Peaks in Menopause, According to ADDitude Reader Survey', Additude magazine, 19 April 2024

35. Jenna Fletcher, 'What are the phases of the menstrual cycle?', Medical News Today, 5 Nov 2019

36. Maxime de Jong, Dora Wynchank and Edwin van Andel, et al., 'Female-specific pharmacotherapy in ADHD: premenstrual adjustment of psychostimulant dosage', Front Psychiatry, vol.14, 13 Dec 2023

37. Ashley Eng, Urveesha Nirjar and Anjeli Elkins, et al., 'Attention-deficit/hyperactivity disorder and the menstrual cycle: Theory and evidence', Hormones and Behavior, Feb 2024; 158:105466

38. Bethan Roberts, Tory Eisenlohr-Moul and Michelle M Martel, 'Reproductive steroids and ADHD symptoms across the menstrual cycle', Journal of Psychoneuroendocrinology, Feb 2018, 88: pp. 105–114

39. ibid

40. ibid

41. Razia Khammissa, Simon Nemutandani and Gal Feller, et al., 'Burnout phenomenon: neurophysiological factors, clinical features, and aspects of management', Journal of International Medical Research, 13 Sept 2022

42. Yugi Higuchi, Masatoshi Inagaki and Toshihiro Koyama, et al., 'A cross-sectional study of psychological distress, burnout, and the associated risk factors in hospital pharmacists in Japan', BMC Public Health, 8 July 2016, 16:534

43. Linda Walker (ADDA Editorial Team), 'ADHD and Burnout in the Workplace: Still Much to Do', Attention Deficit Disorder Association, September 2022

44. Razia Khammissa, Simon Nemutandani and Gal Feller, et al., 'Burnout phenomenon', Journal of International Medical Research, 13 Sept 2022

45. Virginie Mansuy-Aubert and Yann Ravussin, 'Short chain fatty acids: the messengers from down below', Frontiers in Neuroscience, 6 July 2023, vol. 17

46. Kate Moryoussef, 'Rising from ADHD Burnout: A Recovery Kit for Women', Additude magazine blog, 8 Jan 2025

47. Dr. Arielle Schwartz, 'Interoception: A Key to Wellbeing', Center for Resilience Informed Therapy blog, 23 May 2022

48. Seda Kiraz, Sencan Sertçelik and Serap Erdoğan Taycan, 'The Relationship Between Alexithymia and Impulsiveness in Adult Attention Deficit and Hyperactivity Disorder', Turkish Journal of Psychiatry, Summer 2021; 32(2): pp. 109-117

49. Karin Eberhard, 'The effects of visualization on judgment and decision-making', Management Review Quarterly, vol. 73, pp. 167–214 (2023)

50. P Šrámek, M Šimečková and L Janský, et al, 'Human physiological responses to immersion into water of different temperatures', European Journal of Applied Physiology, vol. 81, pp. 436–442 (2000)

51. Dan Pilat and Dr Sekoul Krastev, 'Donald Hebb: Pioneer of Neuropsychology', The Decision Lab, n.d.

52. Tony Robbins on X (formerly Twitter), 'Where focus goes, energy flows', available at: https://x.com/TonyRobbins/status/1536370847555809281

53. 'How Dopamine Influences ADHD Symptoms And Treatment', ADDA (Attention Deficit Disorder Association), 7 Nov 2024

54. Ellen Littman, PhD, 'Never Enough? Why ADHD Brains Crave Stimulation', Additude magazine, 21 August 2024

Resources

Organisations dedicated fully or partially to ADHD

UK

ADHD Foundation, The Neurodiversity Charity (adhdfoundation.org.uk)

Attention Deficit Disorder Information and Support Service (addiss.co.uk)

UK ADHD Partnership (ukadhd.com)

UK Adult ADHD Network (ukaan.org)

USA

American Academy of Child and Adolescent Psychiatry (aacap.org)

American Psychiatric Association (psychiatry.org)

American Psychological Association (apa.org)

Attention Deficit Disorder Association (add.org)

Children and Adults with Attention-Deficit/Hyperactivity Disorder (chadd.org)

Ireland

ADHD Ireland (adhdireland.ie)

Australia

ADHD Support Australia (adhdsupportaustralia.com.au)

ADHD Foundation (adhdfoundation.org.au)

New Zealand

ADHD New Zealand (adhd.org.nz)

Canada

Centre for ADHD Awareness, Canada (caddac.ca)

Web resources

ADHD Women's Wellbeing (adhdwomenswellbeing.co.uk)

ADDConsults (addconsults.com)

ADDitude (additudemag.com)

Faster than Normal (fasterthannormal.com)

How to ADHD (howtoadhd.com; youtube.com/howtoadhd)

Tracy Otsuka (Tracyotsuka.com)

Suggested reading

Barkley, Russell A., and Christine M. Benton PhD, *Taking Charge of Adult ADHD* (Guildford Press, 2010).

Boissiere, Phil, MFT, *Thriving with Adult ADHD: Skills to Strengthen Executive Functioning* (Althea Press, 2018).

Brown, Richard P., MD, and Patricia L. Gerbarg, MD, *Non-Drug Treatments for ADHD: New Options for Kids, Adults, and Clinicians* (W.W. Norton & Company, 2012).

Conner, Alex, and James Brown *ADHD Unpacked: Everything you need to know to survive and thrive as an adult with ADHD* (Bloomsbury, 2025).

Foote, Jeffrey, PhD, Carrie Wilkens, PhD, and Nicole Kosanke, PhD, *Beyond Addiction: How Science and Kindness Help People Change* (New York: Scribner, 2014).

Frates, Beth, MD, Michelle Tollefson, MD, and Amy Comander, MD, *Paving the Path to Wellness Workbook* (Healthy Learning, 2021).

Hallowell, Edward M. MD, *ADHD Explained: Your Toolkit to Understanding and Thriving* (DK, 2023).

Hallowell, Edward M. MD, and John J. Ratey, MD, *ADHD 2.0: New Science and Essential Strategies for Thriving with Distraction from Childhood Through Adulthood* (Ballantine Books, 2021).

Hartmann, Thom, *ADHD: A Hunter in a Farmer's World* (Healing Arts Press, 2019).

Kustow, James, Dr, *How to Thrive with Adult ADHD: 7 Pillars for Focus, Productivity and Balance* (Vermillion, 2024).

Maskell, Leanne, *ADHD an A-Z: Figuring it Out Step by Step* (Jessica Kingsley Publishers, 2022).

Matlen, Terry, MSW, *The Queen of Distraction: How Women with ADHD Can Conquer Chaos, Find Focus, and Get More Done* (New Harbinger Publications, 2014).

Miller, Lucinda, *Brain Brilliance: 60 Nourishing Recipes and a Nutritional Toolkit for Dyslexia, Dyspraxia, ADHD, Autism and all Neurodivergent Kids* (Quadrille Publishing, 2024).

Ramsay, Russel, PhD, *The Adult ADHD and Anxiety Workbook: Cognitive Behavioral Therapy Skills to Manage Stress, Find Focus, and Reclaim Your Life* (New Harbinger, 2024).

Ratey, John J., MD, and Eric Hagerman, *Spark! The Revolutionary New Science of Exercise and the Brain* (Quercus, 2009).

Rosier, Tamara, PhD, *You, Me, and Our ADHD Family: Practical Steps to Cultivate Healthy Relationships* (Revell, 2024).

Rosier, Tamara, PhD, *Your Brain's Not Broken: Strategies for Navigating Your Emotions and Life with ADHD* (Revell, 2021).

Shankman, Peter, *Faster than Normal: Turbocharge Your Focus, Productivity, and Success with the Secrets of the ADHD Brain* (TarcherPerigee, 2017).

Skoglund, Lotta, *ADHD Girls to Women: Getting on The Radar* (Jessica Kingsley Publishers, 2023).

Solden, Sari, MS, and Michelle Frank, PsyD, *A Radical Guide for Women with ADHD: Embrace Neurodiversity, Live Boldy, and Break Through* (New Harbinger Publications, 2019).

Vignola, Nicole, *Rewire: Break the Cycle, Alter Your Thoughts and Create Lasting Change* (Michael Joseph, 2024).

Walker, Matthew, PhD, *Why We Sleep: Unlocking the Power of Sleep and Dreams* (Scribner, 2017).

Zylowska Lidia, MD, *The Mindfulness Prescription for Adult ADHD: An 8-Step Program for Strengthening Attention, Managing Emotions, and Achieving Your Goals* (Trumpeter, 2012).

About the Author

Kate Moryoussef is the host of award-winning and chart-topping The ADHD Women's Wellbeing Podcast, a women's ADHD Lifestyle & Wellbeing Coach, and EFT practitioner. Diagnosed with ADHD at 40, Kate understands firsthand the unique challenges women face in rediscovering their true selves while managing ADHD. With over two decades of experience, she combines insights from her journey, coaching expertise, and qualifications to help newly-diagnosed ADHD women find validation, self-compassion, and authentic empowerment. A mother of four, Kate is passionate about sharing transformative tools that promote calm, confidence, and balance in life, relationships, and work.

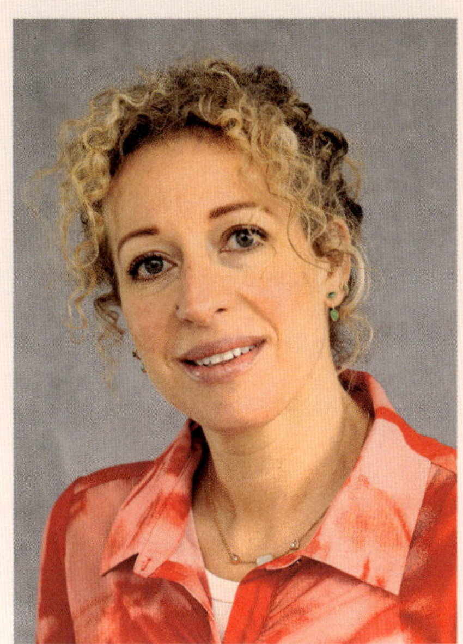

Photography by Ailsa Bee Photography

Acknowledgements

Thank you to my agent, Jessica Killingley, for believing in me and introducing me to my very own book-writing fairy, Lynda Cooper. Lynda, thank you for being the most insightful guardian angel I could wish for. Elizabeth, your guidance has been so gentle yet profound, and Jasmin, you have helped edit and create a book I am truly proud of.

I wouldn't be here without my podcast and the brilliant insights I receive from my guests or my incredible ADHD Women's Wellbeing community – I have adored coaching and learning from you and am so thankful for every minute we spend together.

Thank you to both my parents – your love and support have helped me become who I am today. Words cannot quite express my gratitude to you, Jamie. My rock, my person, my everything. Without your endless patience, morning cups of tea, kindness, love, and belief, this book would never have happened. Lastly, my biggest thanks of all goes to Raph, Ruby, Tali, and Libbie. Everything I do is with you in mind, and I couldn't be prouder of the individuals you are becoming. Loving and supporting you has been the most rewarding job of my life, and I cannot wait to see you all shine.

Publisher's acknowledgements

DK would like to thank Lynda Cooper for editorial support; Kathy Steer for proofreading; the experts for their insightful contributions; and all of the women who kindly shared their ADHD experiences with us.

Disclaimer

Neither the publisher nor the author is engaged in rendering professional advice or services to the individual reader. The ideas, procedures, and suggestions contained in this book are not intended as a substitute for consulting with your doctor or a professional. All matters regarding your health require supervision. Neither the author nor the publisher shall be liable or responsible for any loss or damage allegedly arising from any information or suggestion in this book.

A note on gender identities

DK recognizes all gender identities, and acknowledges that the sex someone was assigned at birth based on their sexual organs may not align with their own gender identity. People may self-identify as any gender or no gender (including, but not limited to, that of a cis or trans woman, of a cis and trans man, or of a non-binary person). As gender language, and its use in our society evolves, scientific and medical communities continue to reassess their own phrasing. Most of the studies referred to in this book use "women" to describe people whose sex was assigned as female at birth and "men" to describe people whose sex was assigned as male at birth.

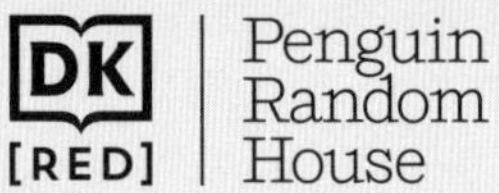

Editorial Director Elizabeth Neep
Editor Jasmin Lennie
Senior Designer Jordan Lambley
Senior Production Editor Tony Phipps
Senior Production Controller Luca Bazzoli
DTP and Design Coordinator Heather Blagden
Jacket Designer Izzy Poulson, Jordan Lambley
Publishing Coordinator Emily Cannings
Art Director Maxine Pedliham
Publishing Director Stephanie Jackson

Design and Illustration Hannah Naughton
Editorial Gaynor Sermon

First published in Great Britain in 2025 by DK RED, an imprint of Dorling Kindersley Limited
20 Vauxhall Bridge Road,
London SW1V 2SA

The authorised representative in the EEA is Dorling Kindersley Verlag GmbH. Arnulfstr. 124, 80636 Munich, Germany

10 9 8 7 6 5 4 3 2 1
001–344795–Jul/2025

A CIP catalogue record for this book is available from the British Library. ISBN: 978-0-2417-1529-1

Printed and bound in China

www.dk.com

This book was made with Forest Stewardship Council™ certified paper – one small step in DK's commitment to a sustainable future.
Learn more at www.dk.com/uk/information/sustainability